Over 200 Low-Fat, Low-Cholesterol,
Low-Salt, Sugar-Free
Divine Vegetarian Entrees, Soups, Salads,

and

Heavenly Healthy Wholegrain
Breads and Desserts
Many Gluten Free Recipes (GF)
Over 65,00 copies sold

THE VEGETARIAN GOURMET

By the authors of Healthy Baking and Mother Nature's Garden

Florence Bienenfeld Ph.D, MFT
Mickey Bienenfeld

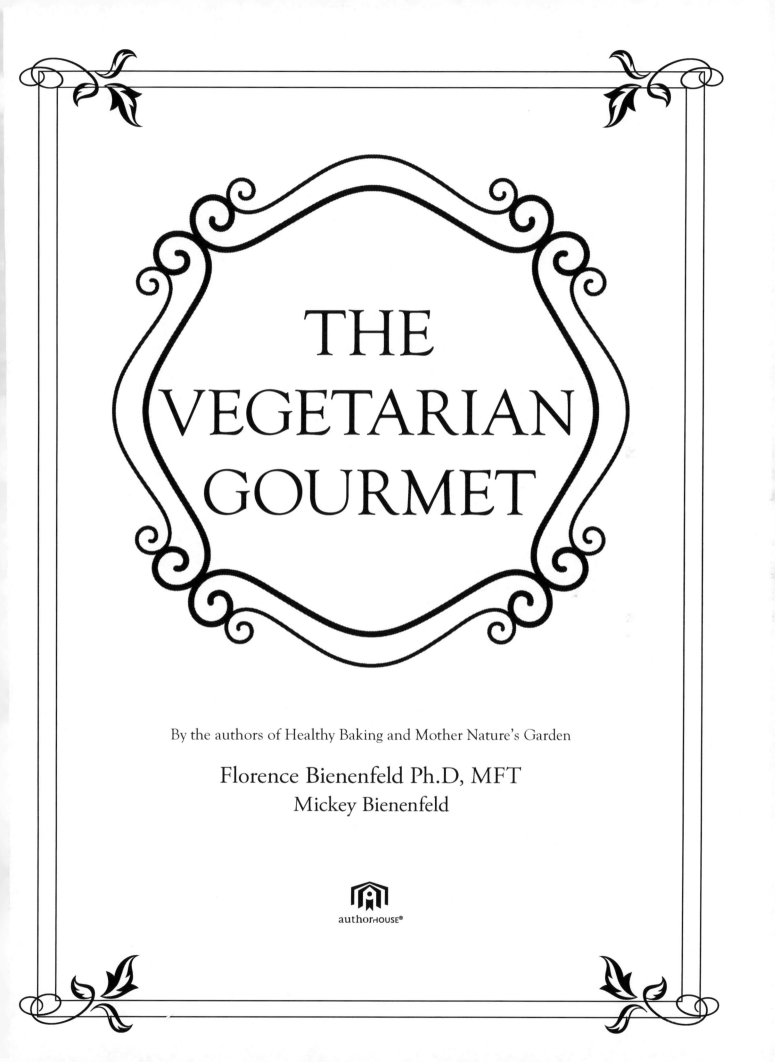
authorHOUSE®

AuthorHouse™ LLC
1663 Liberty Drive
Bloomington, IN 47403
www.authorhouse.com
Phone: 1-800-839-8640

Published by AuthorHouse 05/06/2014

ISBN: 978-1-4918-2971-4 (sc)
ISBN: 978-1-4918-2969-1 (e)

Library of Congress Control Number: 2013919475

ACKNOWLEDGEMENTS

First of all, we wish to thank Joe D. Goldstrich, M.D., F.A.C.C. for his enthusiastic foreword. Dr. Goldstrich is the author of "The Best Chance Diet" (Humanics, 1982, reprinted in 1985); formerly, Cardiologist for Longevity Center in Santa Barbara, California and Director of the Heart Center in Dallas, Texas; and presently in private practice in homeopathy, cardiology and nutrition in Santa Monica, California.

With great love and appreciation, we wish to thank the following family and friends, who have either inspired a particular recipe or have inspired us generally to write this book: Lynn Avins; Ruth and Amanda Barrett; Dodo (Renee) Bienenfeld; Joel Bienenfeld (and Adam); Esther Bienenfeld; Joan Bram; Naomi Enoch; Pamela Juergenson; Joan Kellen; Joan and Michael Lachkar (owners of Michel's Entourage Restaurant, Los Angeles); Sylvia and Ezra Novak; Ellen Rams; Phoebe, Harold, Susan and Karen Reff; Isolina Ricci; Shelly Seltzer; Joy, Elaine and Karen Stelton; Natalie Krol Solomon; Linda Thomas; Charlotte Winokur; and Selma Wities.

We wish to give a very special thank you to Kay Neves, the best typist and friend ever; and also wish to acknowledge Rita Leinwand, a Cordon Bleu and very fine gourmet cooking instructor. Special thanks to Dan Bienenfeld for adjusting and highlighting recipes for Gluten Free eaters.

Another special thank you to James E. Dalen, M.D., Chairman of the Department of Medicine at the University of Massachusetts for reviewing our manuscript and for offering fine suggestions.

FOREWORD

In the United States, approximately 1 million people die each year of heart disease. Approximately 25% of these people die suddenly. Their death is the first sign of their heart disease...the obstructions in their arteries, growing out of a lifetime of eating too much cholesterol and fat.

As a cardiologist, I had seen, only too often, the end stage of this process. When I met Nathan Pritikin in 1977, he assured me that the whole process was almost completely preventable and to some extent, reversable. I became the cardiologist at his Longevity Center in Santa Barbara and later the Medical Director at his center in Santa Monica. I proved to myself that what he said was true. In 1984, the National Heart, Lung and Blood Institute confirmed what Pritikin had been saying and what I had been prescribing as a cardiologist. The facts are in! What you eat does make a difference.

Micky and Flo Bienenfeld's book, while not quite as rigorous as Pritikin, gives you wonderfully delicious recipes to fight off the ravages of cholesterol, fat and blocked arteries. Enjoy, Enjoy, Enjoy.

Joe D. Goldstrich, M.D., F.A.C.C.
Cardiologist and Homeopathic Physician

IMPORTANT INFORMATION AND SUGGESTIONS

1. Read recipe through very carefully before beginning, and assemble all ingredients in recipe. Preheat the oven before baking. Use level measures.

2. Use non-stick baking pans for cakes, cookies, breads and muffins. Fry and saute in non-stick frying pans without oil or fat. (Read instrucions in Appendix.) Use wooden or plastic spoons, spatulas and utensils to avoid scratching non-stick surfaces.

3. Use extra large eggs whenever egg whites are called for. To beat egg whites, start at low speed until whites are foamy, and gradually increase speed to high. If there is any trace of yolk or fat in whites, they will not whip properly.

4. Evaporated skimmed milk comes in cans, which can be purchased or ordered by the case in supermarkets. Double-strength reconstituted non-fat milk powder can be used as a substitute.

5. Whip low-fat cottage cheese in blender or food processor until smooth and creamy, whenever whipped cottage cheese is called for. Avoid boiling soups or sauces after cottage cheese has been added, or cottage cheese will curdle. Avoid overbaking cheesecakes or quiches made with cottage cheese or cottage cheese will curdle.

6. Use whole wheat pastry flour in cakes and breads when it is called for. In the event whole wheat pastry flour is not available in your area, whole wheat flour can be substituted, provided that the amount of flour is reduced by 2 tablespoons per cup. Baking time is increased by 5 to 10 minutes. Always test for doneness. For a moister, slightly heavier texture, use whole wheat flour.

7. Take care not to overbake these low or non-fat/cholesterol cakes and breads, or they become too dry. Remove cakes and breads from the oven as soon as cake tester shows no sign of wet, raw, or unbaked batter. A small crumb of dry batter may still cling to tester. That's O.K. Cakes and breads become a little less moist as they cool.

8. Amount of time required for cooking or baking and number of persons served is only approximate.

9. Be creative and improvise on your own favorite recipes. (Read "How to Improvise on Your Favorite Recipes" in Appendix.)

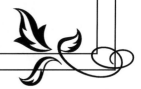

The Introduction

Welcome to enjoying our superb, gourmet, wholesome vegetarian and many Gluten Free recipes. It is a pleasure to share our fun and delicious way of eating with you. We haven't always eaten this way. We used to eat a lot of meat, processed foods and sweets. Our diet was also very rich in cholesterol, fat and salt. We became vegetarians about ten years ago. Then, about five years ago, we decided to reduce our intake of cholesterol, fat and salt, and to avoid sugar, caffein, preservatives and artificial additives entirely from our diet. Our friends are amazed by our energy and vigor and so are we.

It was difficult for us at first, giving up all the foods we knew and loved, until we developed our new marvelous recipes to replace the old ones. Now it feels good to be eating tasty, nourishing foods and tempting sweets that are less rich, but still rich-tasting. For example, our carob brownies taste delicious, yet they contain only 1 tablespoon of oil, instead of 1 cup of oil or butter per recipe. Do you know that a cup of oil or butter contains 1600 calories?

We sometimes share a whole creamy custard pie without guilt or a heavy feeling afterwards, because it is made of evaporated skimmed milk, egg whites, a little honey and vanilla. We can munch on our wholesome crunchy and chewy cookies to our hearts delight and feel self-righteous. These contain a variety of wholegrain cereals, egg whites, honey or fruit juice, raisins, carob and spices.

Our easy-to-prepare recipes are original. They contain only the purest, most natural wholegrain and unprocessed ingredients. They are also very low in fat, cholesterol and salt. We throw the yolks of the eggs away and use only the whites. We use non-fat and low-fat dairy products. We avoid both white and brown sugar, white flour and products containing salt, preservatives and additives of any sort. Many of the recipes are already Gluten Free, or can be converted to be.

We try to use as little sweetening as possible in our recipes. In some of our dessert recipes only fruit juice or fruit is used. We use honey instead of sugar because honey is an unprocessed food, complete with all of its own natural enzymes. We do not experience the "sugar low" we used to get with the small amounts of fruit juice and honey we eat.

Every once in a while we will taste rich food or desserts, but it tastes too rich or too sweet for us. What fun it is to be able to enjoy our lean, wholesome and pure cooking and baking. Our friends and family enthusiastically enjoy the delicious and nutritious foods and desserts we have created. They love to dine with us.

So enjoy preparing our recipes and eating our superb gourmet vegetarian cooking and baking. We wish you all bon appetit.

Florence and Mickey Bienenfeld

DEDICATION

To the many millions of men and women
who choose to reduce their fat, cholesterol, gluten,
salt and sugar intake; and to all who wish to enjoy superb,
nutritious, gourmet, vegetarian cooking and baking at its finest.

THE CONTENTS

Foreword, vii

Important Information And Suggestions, ix

The Introduction, xi

Breakfast & Brunch, 1

Soups & Breads, 17

Salads & Dressings, 41

Main Courses, 55

Desserts, 111

Potpourri, 159

Basic Recipes, 181

BREAKFAST & BRUNCH

Breakfast is a very important meal. A hearty, wholesome breakfast can get you off to a good start, and give you and your loved ones the energy you all need for a productive day. It is so sad to see so many people beginning their day with a donut, coffee and a cigarette.

Breakfast time is the perfect time to eat whole grains which provide Vitamins B, and E and roughage for your body. Brunch is a delightful way to entertain friends. This section offers you a variety of exciting, healthful and tasty breakfast and brunch recipes, which are low in salt, fat and cholesterol. So here's wishing you a really good day, every day!

Stuffed Papaya Halves Indian (GF)

This delicate dish is really different. Your guests won't stop raving.

2 cups low-fat cottage cheese
3 tablespoons potato starch, or cornstarch
2 tablespoons honey
1 tablespoon rum (optional)
1 ¼ teaspoons curry powder
⅛ teaspoon chili powder
1/16 teaspoon cayenne
½ teaspoon ground coriander
¼ teaspoon cinnamon

¼ cup raisins

3 ripe Hawaiian papayas, halved and seeded

sprinkle of coriander for topping

Mix together first 9 ingredients in a food processor or blender until smooth. Stir in raisins. Fill 6 papaya halves, sprinkle tops with coriander, and place them in a 9x13-inch non-stick or glass oven-proof baking pan. Bake in a 450° oven for 15 minutes only. Do not overbake. Serve hot. Serves 4 to 6.

Hot Cracked Wheat, Oats and Bran Cereal

For a healthy, delicious hot cereal, mix equal parts of cracked wheat and rolled oats, then add 2 tablespoons or more of unprocessed bran for each cup of cereal mixture. Store in an air-tight container in the refrigerator.

1 cup Cracked Wheat-Oats-Bran Cereal mixture
2 cups water

Continues on the next page

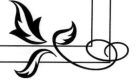

Mix together cereal and water in a small non-stick saucepan. Bring cereal to a boil, reduce heat, and cook for 8 to 10 minutes. Serves 2.

Note: — Serve cooked cereal with non-fat milk, honey, sunflower seeds and raisins.

Healthy Seven Grain and Bran Cereal

For a healthy and hearty hot cereal, mix equal parts of 7-grain cereal and rolled oats. Add 2 tablespoons or more of unprocessed bran to each cup of mixture, as desired. Store mixture in an airtight container in refrigerator.

1 cup Seven Grain and Bran Cereal mixture
2 cups water

Mix cereal and water together in a small, non-stick pan. Bring cereal to boil, reduce heat, and cook for 8 to 10 minutes. Serves 2.

Note: — Serve with non-fat milk and honey, if desired. Sunflower seeds and raisins are also nice.

Pumpkin-Spiced Cereal

This spicy cereal is an exciting change and especially fun and warming on a cold morning. Leftovers can be eaten as a snack pudding.

½ cup whole grain cereal, uncooked
½ cup evaporated skimmed milk
¾ cup water
1 cup canned pumpkin
½ teaspoon cinnamon
½ teaspoon allspice
¼ teaspoon coriander

Continues on the next page

2 tablespoons black raisins

1 to 2 tablespoons honey

Cook all ingredients in a non-stick saucepan over medium heat. Stir occasionally for approximately 10 minutes, or until mixture thickens and cereal is ready to serve. Serves 2.

Buckwheat Kernel Cereal

Serve this hearty cereal with honey if desired. Buckwheat has the highest protein value of any grain. Seed meal and granular lecithin may be added to boost nutrition, and give the cereal a nutty flavor.

1 cup Roasted Buckwheat Kernels (Kasha)

1 egg white

2 teaspoons onion powder

¼ teaspoon ground pepper

2 cups boiling water

In a small mixing bowl mix together buckwheat kernels, egg white and onion powder, and mix until kernels are well coated. Fry the kernels in a non-stick frying pan turning frequently until kernels are dry, then cook mixture in a saucepan with the boiling water and pepper until water is absorbed, for approximately 5 to 8 minutes. Serves 2.

Scrambled Egg Whites, Onions & Tomatoes Ranchero (GF)

Who says we can't have eggs ranchero the low cholesterol way? Here is how to do it.

1 tablespoon water

½ medium onion, cut in bite-size pieces

Continues on the next page

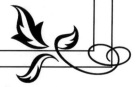

1 green onion, chopped
2 medium tomatoes, cut in bite-size pieces

6 egg whites
2 tablespoons evaporated skimmed milk
½ teaspoon chili powder

In a large non-stick frying pan saute onion in water until golden brown. Stir in green onion and tomatoes and cook until moisture is absorbed, stirring occasionally.

Whisk egg whites, milk and chili powder until frothy. Stir egg white mixture into sauteed vegetables in frying pan. Scramble until desired consistency. Serves 2.

Individual Egg White Cheese Omelette with Herbs (GF)

This omelette tastes really gourmet, and has very little cholesterol. Use chopped fresh herbs whenever possible.

½ teaspoon onion powder
⅓ cup low-fat cottage cheese

3 egg whites
pinch of oregano
pinch of basil
pinch of thyme
1 tablespoon chopped parsley

Mix together onion powder and cottage cheese and set aside. In a small bowl beat egg whites and herbs with a fork and fry this mixture in a hot, lightly greased non-stick omelette pan until set on one side. Then turn and fry for a few seconds on the other side. Quickly spread cottage cheese mixture on ½ of omelette, fold omelette over, and fry on both sides until cottage cheese is warm and begins to melt. Turn onto a warm plate and serve at once. Serves 1.

Note: — For a gourmet mushroom-cheese omelette prepare the egg whites as directed. Instead of filling it with cottage cheese, fill it with hot Mushroom-Cheese Sauce, and serve immediately.

Low-Fat Cheese Blintzes

Serve *these* wholesome, delicious blintzes with Mock Sour Cream and fresh fruit or with Flo's Homemade Orange Marmalade. For a special treat make blintzes into a Blintze Souffle. (See recipe below.)

2 pounds hoop cheese (a dry skimmed milk cheese)
½ cup evaporated skimmed milk (or non-fat milk if desired)
4 tablespoons honey
1 teaspoon cinnamon
1 teaspoon coriander
2 teaspoons lemon juice

1 teaspoon grated lemon rind

12 to 14 Tender Whole Wheat Crepes or Whole Wheat Crepes Without Milk
    (see chapter on Basics)

Mix together first 7 ingredients in blender or food processor until well blended. Fill each crepe with a generous, heaping tablespoon of cheese mixture, and roll up crepes. Ends may be left open or folded under as desired. Fry in a non-stick frying pan until brown on both sides and heated through. Yields 12 to 14 blintzes.

Blintze Souffle

To prepare Blintze Souffle: Arrange unfried blintzes in a 9x13-inch non-stick or glass oven-proof baking pan. Prepare 1 recipe of Vanilla Custard Pie (see Index). Pour custard over blintzes and bake in a 350° oven for 25 minutes, or just until custard is set. Do not overbake. Serve warm. Serves 6 to 8.

Custard Noodle Pudding with Orange Peel & Spices

This noodle pudding has a wonderful flavor and makes an excellent brunch or buffet dish.

⅔ cup honey

2 cups low-fat cottage cheese, whipped

1 ½ cups evaporated skimmed milk

1 cup water

1 teaspoon grated orange rind, or Cooked Orange Peel (see chapter on Basics)

8 egg whites

1 ½ teaspoons vanilla extract

2 tablespoons whole wheat pastry flour

¼ teaspoon coriander

⅛ teaspoon cardamom

1 cup black raisins

12 ounces whole wheat noodles, cooked, rinsed in cold water, drained

sprinkle of nutmeg over top before baking

Whisk together first 10 ingredients in a large mixing bowl. Stir in raisins and noodles. Spread mixture in a 9x13-inch non-stick or glass oven-proof baking pan. Sprinkle generously with nutmeg. Bake in a 350° oven for 45 to 50 minutes, or until lightly brown, and knife comes out clean 1 ½ inches from the center. Cool for 15 minutes before serving, or serve cold. Serves 10 to 12.

Flo's Fabulous French Toast (GF)

This recipe combines whole grain bread or Gluten free bread, milk and egg whites to create a sustaining complete protein breakfast food, for you and your family. Top with honey, pure maple syrup, or Flo's Homemade Orange Marmalade, and serve with Hot Carob-Postum Drink and fresh fruit. I recently prepared this while camping in Sequoia, and was it ever delicious!

¾ cup evaporated skimmed milk
6 egg whites
1 teaspoon cinnamon
1 tablespoon honey

6 slices soft whole wheat bread or Gluten free bread, cut ½-inch thick

Whisk the first 4 ingredients in a small mixing bowl until well beaten. Pour milk-egg white mixture into a shallow pie plate, and soak slices of bread on both sides. Fry in a non-stick griddle or frying pan until lightly brown on both sides, but moist inside. Do not overcook. Serves 4 to 6.

Divine Apple Crepes

These apple crepes taste delicious on their own. For a special treat serve them with Honey Vanilla Sauce.

6 red or golden Delicious apples, unpeeled, sliced
1 ½ teaspoons cinnamon
⅓ cup concentrated apple juice
1 handful of chopped walnuts (optional)
1 handful of black raisins

12 to 14 Whole Wheat Tender Crepes (see chapter on Basics)

sprinkle of cinnamon

Continues on the next page

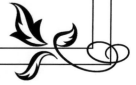

Saute first 5 ingredients in a large non-stick frying pan until apples are tender. Stir frequently until most of the moisture is absorbed. Spread hot apple slices on one side of each crepe, fold the other side over and sprinkle top with cinnamon. Heat filled crepes in a non-stick 10x15-inch jelly roll pan in a 400° oven for 10 to 15 minutes, just until heated through. Yields 12 to 14 crepes.

Buckwheat Hotcakes

Buckwheat flour is very high in protein, especially when combined with dairy products and egg whites. You will love the flavor topped with honey, maple syrup, or Black Raisin Syrup.

2 tablespoons non-fat yogurt
1 cup non-fat milk, less 2 tablespoons
1 tablespoon blackstrap molasses
1 tablespoon pure maple syrup
½ teaspoon vanilla
1 egg white

1 cup buckwheat flour
1 teaspoon baking soda

Whisk first 6 ingredients in a mixing bowl. Mix together flour and soda, and add, all at once, whisking just until smooth. Fry pancakes on a hot non-stick griddle until brown on both sides. Serves 2.

Non-Dairy Apple Pancakes

A luscious non-dairy treat, and sweetened only with apple juice!

½ cup cold water
3 tablespoons concentrated apple juice
1 teaspoon vanilla extract

Continues on the next page

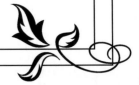

1 teaspoon lemon juice
8 egg whites
1 cup whole wheat flour
1 teaspoon baking powder

2 apples, peeled and cut into ¼-inch slices
¼ cup concentrated apple juice
1 tablespoon cinnamon

pure maple syrup (optional)

Whisk the first 5 ingredients in a large mixing bowl. Mix together flour and baking powder and add, all at once, whisking just until smooth.

Saute apple slices with apple juice and cinnamon in 6-inch non-stick pan or omelette pan over medium-high heat, stirring until golden brown.

Remove ½ of apples from the pan. Pour ½ of batter over apples left in the pan, and cook on one side until set, for about 2 minutes. Slide pancake onto a large plate, hold skillet over pancake, and invert pancake back into skillet. Fry until underside is set, for about 2 minutes. Slide pancake into a non-stick baking pan and set aside. Prepare second pancake. Sprinkle with cinnamon, and bake pancakes in a 400° oven for 5 minutes. Serve immediately. Serves 2.

Fat-Free Passover Pancakes (GF)

These Passover pancakes are delicious all year round. Serve with a few drops of honey.

4 egg whites
½ cup non-fat milk
½ cup apple juice
½ teaspoon cinnamon
¾ cup finely ground whole wheat or Gluten free matza crumbs – or Passover cake meal

Whisk first 4 ingredients in a medium-sized mixing bowl. Add matza crumbs, or cake meal and beat just until blended. Drop tablespoonfuls of batter in a hot, non-stick frying pan, and fry until brown on both sides. Serves 2.

Blueberry Pancakes

These pancakes are a special treat.

2 tablespoons honey
1 teaspoon cinnamon
2 cups non-fat milk
2 egg whites
1 tablespoon lemon juice
¼ teaspoon vanilla

2 cups whole wheat flour
4 teaspoons baking powder

1 cup fresh or frozen blueberries

Whisk the first 6 ingredients in a medium-size mixing bowl. Mix together flour and baking powder, and add, all at once, whisking just until blended. Do not overbeat. Gently fold in blueberries.

Heat a non-stick griddle or frying pan. Pour ¼ cup batter for each pancake. Turn over once. Serve with pure maple syrup, or honey if desired. Serves 2 or 3.

Individual Cottage Cheese Pancake

This pancake is nutritious, and a delightful way to start the day.

⅓ cup low-fat cottage cheese
1 egg white
2 tablespoons whole wheat flour
¼ teaspoon cinnamon
1 teaspoon concentrated apple juice
sprinkle of cinnamon

1 teaspoon concentrated apple juice for topping

Continues on the next page

Beat together first 6 ingredients with a fork until combined. Heat a non-stick lightly greased omelette pan. Fry pancake over medium-low heat until set, and brown on one side. Loosen very carefully, turn it over, and spread 1 teaspoon apple juice on top. Fry until puffed and brown on other side.

Serve at once with a sprinkle of cinnamon. Serves 1.

Carmelized Apple Pancakes

Such a treat is hard to beat!

Apple Topping:
4 cups thinly sliced tart green apples, unpeeled
⅓ cup concentrated apple juice
2 teaspoons cinnamon

Pancake Batter:
2 tablespoons honey
1 teaspoon cinnamon
1 ½ cups non-fat milk
2 egg whites
1 scant tablespoon lemon juice
¼ teaspoon vanilla

1 ½ cups whole wheat flour
1 tablespoon baking powder

Topping:
2 tablespoons concentrated apple juice, honey, or maple syrup sprinkle of cinnamon

To prepare Apple Topping: Saute apple slices, apple juice and 2 teaspoons cinnamon in a 10-inch non-stick frying pan until apples are tender and apple juice becomes syrupy. Set aside.

To prepare Pancake Batter: Meanwhile prepare the pancake batter: Whisk the first 6 ingredients into a mixing bowl, until well mixed. Mix together flour and baking powder, and add, all at once, whisking just until blended. Do not overbeat.

Continues on the next page

To assemble Apple Pancake: Preheat broiler. Remove ½ of the apple slices from pan, and reserve them for the second pancake. Spread apple slices left in the pan evenly. Heat the pan and pour ½ of the batter on top of the apple slices. Fry pancake over medium-high heat, until brown on the bottom, and pancake bubbles and begins to shrink away from sides of pan. Loosen bottom all around with a spatula. Place a large dinner plate on top of the pan, turn pancake over onto the plate, then slide it back into the pan. Cook until bottom side is brown. Remove pancake from pan and repeat process, or both pancakes can be made at the same time in 2 separate non-stick frying pans. Set both pancakes in a 10x15-inch non-stick jelly roll pan.

Spread apple juice, honey or maple syrup on top of each pancake, and sprinkle each pancake generously with cinnamon. Place pancakes under broiler for a few minutes until bubbly. Serve at once. Serves 2 or 3.

Passover Apple-Raisin-Nut Souffle with Honey-Wine Sauce

This delicious souffle is a real treat on Passover or at any time, and especially when served with Honey-Wine Sauce.

8 egg whites
½ cup Passover cake meal

2 cups grated sweet apples, cored and unpeeled
½ cup chopped nuts
¼ cup sweet red wine, or apple juice
2 teaspoons cinnamon

sprinkle of cinnamon for top

Beat egg whites until foamy in an electric mixer. Add cake meal and continue beating on high speed until whites are stiff. Fold in remaining ingredients by hand. Sprinkle with cinnamon.

Bake in a 9x9-inch non-stick or glass oven-proof baking pan for 35 minutes, or until light brown. Serve warm or cold with Honey-Wine Sauce. Serves 6.

Honey-Wine Sauce (GF)

8 egg whites
½ cup honey
⅓ cup sweet white wine
2 cups non-fat milk
⅓ cup potato starch

Whisk all ingredients together in a mixing bowl until foamy. Pour into a non-stick saucepan, and heat until mixture thickens. Cool, blend until smooth in a blender or food processor, and store sauce in the refrigerator. Makes 1-quart of sauce.

Fat-Free Passover Matza Brei (GF)

3 whole wheat matza or Gluten free matza

½ cup apple juice
½ teaspoon cinnamon

6 egg whites, lightly beaten

Break matza into small pieces in a large mixing bowl. Stir in apple juice and cinnamon and soak for 5 minutes. Meanwhile whisk egg whites in another bowl until frothy, and add them to matza mixture. Pour mixture in a hot, non-stick frying pan, and fry matza brei until brown on both sides. Serves 2 to 3.

SOUPS & BREADS

Soups & Breads

Hot and Hearty Soups and Cold Soups,
Plus Marvelous Breads and Muffins

In this section you will find flavorful mushroom-barley soup, minestrone soup, bean soups, lentil soups, creamy vegetable soups, spicy soups, mild soothing soups, and cold refreshing soups—all with little or no fat, cholesterol or salt.

If these soups sound good, wait until you enjoy these hearty soups with tasty, hot, moist homemade breads and muffins, all made without egg yolks, shortening, butter, oil, sugar or salt.

Soups and breads are easy to prepare, inexpensive to serve and nourishing meals in themselves. Leftover soups can be stored in the refrigerator for several days, or frozen for further use.

Wholegrain breads should be stored in the refrigerator or freezer and taken out as needed.

Creamy Lentil-Potato Soup (GF)

This warming soup will fill you up in such a satisfying way. It's a meal in itself.

2 cups raw lentils
6 cups water

3 medium boiling potatoes, cut in large chunks
1 large onion, cut in quarters
4 cloves garlic, whole
2 large stalks celery, sliced thick (approximately 1 cup)
½ cup parsley leaves
2 large carrots (or 4 small carrots), whole
1 tablespoon basil
2 bay leaves
⅓ teaspoon pepper

2 teaspoons onion powder
2 cups low-fat cottage cheese, whipped

garnish of chopped parsley or green onions

Bring lentils and water to a boil in a large soup pot over high heat while you prepare vegetables. Stir in next 9 ingredients. After mixture comes to a boil, cover, reduce heat to medium-low and cook for approximately 1 ½ hours, or until lentils are tender. Puree lentils and vegetables in batches in a food processor or blender and return to the soup pot. Before serving stir in whipped cottage cheese and onion powder and heat soup to just below boiling point. Do not boil. Garnish and serve. Serves 6.

Thick Spicy Lentil Soup (GF)

This hearty, satisfying soup can stay for a week in the refrigerator or may be frozen in quart jars until ready for use. When served with great tasting Homemade Fat-Free and Salt-Free Corn Bread you will be enjoying a completely balanced, nutritious meal.

2 ½ cups uncooked lentils, rinsed
1 cup tomato puree
9 cups water
1 tablespoon red wine vinegar
1 tablespoon chili powder
¼ teaspoon black pepper
1 tablespoon onion powder
½ teaspoon garlic powder
2 bay leaves

6 carrots, sliced
4 long stalks of celery, sliced
½ red or green bell pepper, chopped
1 large onion, chopped
4 Summer squash (or 2 zucchini or crookneck squash), sliced
1 parsnip, whole
4 cups chopped tomatoes (or an additional cup of tomato puree)
1 cup fresh or frozen okra, sliced

Bring the first 9 ingredients to a boil in a large covered soup pot and cook over medium-low heat for 1 hour, stirring occasionally to avoid sticking and burning.

Meanwhile prepare vegetables. When lentils are tender add vegetables and bring soup to boil again. Lower heat and simmer soup for another hour or until vegetables are tender.

To prepare this soup in a large crockpot: Mix all ingredients together in the morning, turn temperature to high and let soup cook until dinnertime. Serves 6 to 8.

Thick Minestrone Soup (GF)

This recipe makes a large pot of delicious and wholesome soup. Serve with raisin Gluten Free Bread. It couldn't be healthier.

½ cup dried pink beans
½ cup dried pinto beans
½ cup dried garbanzo beans
½ cup dried northern white beans
½ cup dried red beans
½ cup dried lima beans
9 cups water

5 cups water
2 bay leaves

1 large onion, finely chopped
3 cloves garlic, minced
2 cups chopped celery and leaves

6 medium tomatoes, chopped
¼ cup minced parsley
¼ teaspoon ground pepper
2 teaspoons Italian seasonings

6 zucchini sliced
2 cups shredded cabbage

2 tablespoons red wine vinegar or apple cider vinegar

Bring beans and 9 cups of water to a boil in a large soup pot and cook over high heat for 10 minutes, remove from heat and allow beans to remain in hot water until cool or overnight. Rinse beans and return to pot.

Cook the beans in 5 cups of water with bay leaves for 2 hours. Saute onion, garlic and celery in a non-stick frying pan until brown, adding a little water, if needed. Add these sauteed vegetables to the beans along with the tomatoes, parsley, pepper and herbs. Simmer covered for 25 minutes. Then add the cabbage and squash (and additional water if a thinner soup is desired). Continue cooking until cabbage and squash are just tender. Add vinegar and serve. Serves 8 to 10.

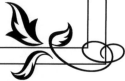

Mushroom Barley Bean Soup

This hearty soup provides a complete wholesome meal in itself. It is especially good on a cold winter's night.

2 cups large sized, dried lima beans
water to cover

6 cups water
1 medium onion, chopped
¼ cup parsley leaves, chopped (or 2 teaspoons dried parsley flakes)
½ tablespoon chopped fresh dill (or ½ teaspoon dried dill weed)
¼ teaspoon black pepper
½ teaspoon celery seed

½ cup barley

3 carrots, sliced
3 stalks celery, sliced
5 large fresh mushrooms or 10 smaller ones, chopped

1 tablespoon fresh parsley (or 1 teaspoon dried parsley flakes)
½ tablespoon fresh chopped dill (or ½ teaspoon dried dill weed)
½ teaspoon celery seed
⅛ teaspoon black pepper
¼ teaspoon garlic powder
1 teaspoon onion powder
1 tablespoon apple cider vinegar or red wine vinegar

Bring the beans and water to a boil in a soup pot and cook for 10 minutes. Turn off heat and allow beans to remain in hot water until cool or overnight. Rinse beans and return them to pot.

To prepare soup on the stove: Stir in next 6 ingredients to the pot and cook beans, covered, very slowly, for approximately 2 to 2 ½ hours or until almost tender. Add the barley and simmer for 1 hour longer. One-half hour before serving add the carrots, celery and mushrooms and 10 minutes before serving add all the remaining 7 ingredients. Serve soup topped with a sprinkle of dill. Serves 6 to 8.

Continues on the next page

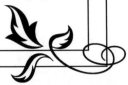

Note: — To prepare soup in a crockpot: Follow instructions in the first paragraph above, place rinsed beans in crockpot and stir in next 10 ingredients. Cook on the highest setting for 8 to 10 hours, then add last 7 ingredients 10 to 15 minutes before serving.

Cold Cucumber-Dill Soup (GF)

This is a lovely cooling soup perfect for summer. Usually cucumber soups are made with cream, butter and salt, but not ours. You won't even miss it.

2 ½ medium cucumbers, peeled, cut lengthwise, seeded

½ cup water
3 teaspoons onion powder
½ teaspoon celery seed
¼ teaspoon ground white pepper (or black)

1 tablespoon fresh dill, chopped
1 green onion, chopped
½ cup buttermilk

1 cup buttermilk
1 teaspoon lemon juice (or more as desired)
2 teaspoons apple cider vinegar

Peel and seed cucumbers. Reserve ½ cucumber. Cut 2 cucumbers into pieces and place pieces in a medium-sized saucepan. Stir in next 4 ingredients, and cook until cucumber is tender and liquid is almost gone, for approximately 20 to 30 minutes. Cool slightly, then puree mixture in a blender or food processor and pour mixture into a medium-sized bowl. Puree reserved half of raw cucumber, dill, green onion and ½ cup of the buttermilk until smooth. Stir into cooked cucumber mixture along with additional cup of buttermilk, lemon and vinegar to taste.

Refrigerate until serving. Serves 2 or 3.

Note: — Buttermilk can be poured through cheesecloth to remove traces of butterfat if desired. If you plan to double the recipe, use only ¾ cup of water instead of 1 cup.

Creamy French Onion Soup (GF)

This marvelous soup makes a great lunch or dinner entree. It is nutritious, tasty and filling. Serve with a green salad or fresh fruit salad.

4 large Spanish onions, sliced
2 tablespoons sherry or semi-sweet white wine
3 cloves garlic

2 cups water
2 cups Cauliflower Broth (see chapter on Basics)

1 ½ cups evaporated skimmed milk

1 cup low-fat cottage cheese
¼ teaspoon black pepper or white pepper

4 thick slices of soft wholegrain or Gluten Free bread or rolls (½-inch thick), sprinkled with
    onion powder and garlic powder and toasted on both sides in the oven

Saute onions, garlic and wine in a large soup pot over medium heat until onions have softened and moisture is absorbed. Puree onions and return to pot. Add cauliflower broth and water. Bring onion soup to boil, cover and cook for one hour, stirring occasionally.

Just before serving add milk to the soup and return it to a boil. Lower flame and stir in cottage cheese and pepper until cottage cheese melts. Serve with a slice of toasted bread in each bowl. Serves 4 to 6.

Note: — *This soup can be made the day before up to the point of adding the cheese. Add cheese just before heating either on the stove, or under the broiler in individual bowls, with a slice of toasted bread in each bowl. Heat until soup is bubbly hot and golden brown.*

Easy Split Pea Soup with Dill (GF)

This recipe makes a hearty, complete protein meal when combined with whole grain bread or rolls.

2 ½ cups split peas
8 cups water
1 medium large onion, cut into quarters
¼ cup fresh parsley (or 1 tablespoon dried parsley)
2 tablespoons fresh dill weed, chopped (or 1 tablespoon dried dill weed)
2 stalks celery, cut into pieces (or 1 tablespoon celery seeds)

2 tablespoons whole wheat pastry or Gluten Free flour
¼ cup cold water

1 10-ounce package frozen peas and carrots
2 teaspoons wine vinegar
2 teaspoons onion powder
¼ teaspoon black pepper
1 teaspoon dried dill weed

Bring the first 6 ingredients to a boil in a large covered soup pot, lower heat and simmer for 1 to 1 ¼ hours or until split peas are very tender. Dissolve flour in ¼ cup of water, add flour mixture to soup, and stir as soup thickens. Remove from heat and cool a little. Puree mixture and return it to soup pot.

Stir in peas and carrots, vinegar and spices. Heat soup slowly, stirring frequently for approximately 15 to 20 minutes or until soup comes to a boil and vegetables are barely tender. Serves 6.

Easy Lima Bean Soup (GF)

For a delicious meal serve this hearty and healthy soup with Homemade Fat-Free and Salt-Free Banana Bread or Gluten Free Bread.

2 cups dried lima beans
6 cups water

4 cups water
1 large onion
½ teaspoon ground pepper
1 teaspoon dried dill weed
1 teaspoon thyme
2 medium tomatoes, chopped

1 10-ounce package frozen baby lima beans, thawed
1 10-ounce package frozen peas and carrots, thawed
2 tablespoons red wine vinegar or apple cider vinegar

Bring beans and 6 cups of water to boil in a large soup pot and cook over high heat for 10 minutes. Remove from heat and allow beans to remain in hot water until cool or overnight. Rinse beans and return them to pot.

Cook beans with the next 6 ingredients in a large crockpot for 10 hours on highest temperature, or in a covered soup pot on the stove for 2 ½ hours or until beans are tender. Add frozen thawed vegetables and vinegar during the last 10 to 15 minutes of cooking. Serves 6.

Easy Lentil-Vegetable Soup (GF)

This easy-to-prepare soup makes a hearty, nutritious meal, especially when served with Whole Wheat Orange-Raisin Rolls or Gluten Free Bread. The combination of lentils and grains provides as much protein as a meat meal.

Continues on the next page

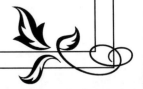

2 cups brown lentils

8 cups boiling water

2 medium tomatoes, cut in small pieces

2 cups okra, cut in pieces

1 medium onion, diced

4 carrots, sliced

4 stalks of celery, sliced

2 cloves of garlic, chopped

8 sprigs of parsley

2 bay leaves

¼ teaspoon black pepper

2 teaspoons Italian seasonings

1 teaspoon celery seed

1 teaspoon onion powder

1 teaspoon dill weed

Bring the first 10 ingredients to a boil in a large covered pot and cook until lentils and vegetables are soft, for approximately 1 ½ hours, or cook slowly in crockpot on highest temperature for the entire day. Ten minutes before serving add the remaining 5 ingredients. Serves 6.

Thick Indian Lentil Soup (GF)

This exotically flavored soup makes an exciting complete protein meal in itself.

2 cups raw lentils

3 cups Cauliflower Broth (see chapter on Basics)

3 cups water

1 large tomato

1 clove garlic

3 to 4 dates, pitted

Continues on the next page

¾ teaspoon ground ginger
1 ¼ teaspoons dry mustard
1 tablespoon cumin
1 tablespoon curry powder
1 ½ cups water

1 ½ cups evaporated skimmed milk

Cook lentils in Cauliflower Broth and water until tender. Allow lentils to cool a little, puree them, and return them to the soup pot. Puree tomato, garlic and dates and add this mixture to pureed lentils. Stir in spices and water, and simmer soup slowly for 20 minutes. Add evaporated skimmed milk, then heat and serve. Serves 4 to 6.

Creamy Tomato Soup with Herbs

The combination of this delightful soup and the spicy bread is bound to warm the cockles of your heart and your stomach.

3 cups tomato puree
3 cups water
1 tablespoon onion powder
½ teaspoon celery seed
1 teaspoon parsley
1 teaspoon dried basil, crumbled
¼ teaspoon ground pepper
½ teaspoon honey

2 or 3 tablespoons whole wheat pastry flour
1 cup evaporated skimmed milk

Heat first 8 ingredients in a covered soup pot until mixture boils. Reduce heat and simmer for 45 minutes over medium-low heat. In a small mixing bowl mix milk and flour together until smooth. Stir in 1 cup of the hot tomato mixture, then slowly stir milk-flour mixture into the pot of tomato soup until soup thickens slightly. If soup should curdle, beat in blender until smooth, then heat again and serve. Serves 4.

Hearty Lentil-Barley Soup with Vegetables

This soup has excellent flavor and high protein food value. It is a hearty soup, very economical and nourishing.

2 ¼ cups raw lentils, rinsed (1 pound)
11 cups water

½ cup barley
3 bay leaves

2 cups chopped cauliflower
2 cups chopped broccoli
2 cups sliced carrots
1 cup sliced celery
1 medium onion, chopped
2 tablespoons fresh chopped parsley

1 teaspoon celery seed
2 teaspoons dill weed
¼ teaspoon black pepper
2 tablespoons vinegar

Bring lentils and water to boil in a large covered soup pot. Stir in barley and bay leaves and simmer mixture for ½ hour, then add the chopped and sliced vegetables. Return pot to full boil, reduce heat and simmer soup for approximately 45 minutes to 1 hour or until lentils are tender. Add spices and vinegar the last 10 minutes and serve. Makes 10 to 12 hearty servings.

Creamy Potato-Leeks Soup (GF)

This lovely, warming soup makes a nourishing meal all by itself. You are bound to want seconds.

3 leeks, white parts only
6 to 8 celery stalks
3 boiling potatoes

1 cup Garbanzo Broth or Cauliflower Broth (see chapter on Basics), or vegetable broth

3 cups non-fat milk (or 1 ½ cups evaporated skimmed milk and 1 ½ cups water)

1 ⅔ cups low-fat cottage cheese, whipped
⅛ teaspoon cayenne
⅛ teaspoon black pepper

chopped green onions or chives for garnish

Slice vegetables in food processor or cut into thin slices by hand. Saute vegetables over medium-high heat in a non-stick Dutch oven, or stainless steel, or enamel soup pot for 10 minutes. Stir occasionally to keep vegetables from sticking and burning. Add bean or vegetable broth, cover and cook slowly for approximately 20 minutes or until vegetables are soft. Puree the vegetables, then return the pureed vegetables to the pot. Just before serving add milk and return soup to a boil. Lower flame and stir in cottage cheese and seasonings until cottage cheese melts. Do not boil. Serve with a garnish of chopped green onions. Serves 4.

Beet Borscht with Boiled Potatoes (GF)

This is a healthy refreshing soup for summer time, or for anytime.

1 bunch beets, peeled, cooked in 6 cups of water until tender, drained, broth reserved
2 cups beet broth
2 teaspoons onion powder
½ teaspoon black pepper
4 tablespoons red wine vinegar

Continues on the next page

2 tablespoons concentrated apple juice

4 tablespoons low-fat cottage cheese

2 tablespoons non-fat yogurt

4 cups beet broth

4 to 6 boiled potatoes, hot, peeled, whole

Puree first 8 ingredients in a blender or food processor just until beets are grated. Pour mixture into a large-sized mixing bowl and stir in remaining beet broth. Serve chilled with a hot boiled potato in each bowl. Serves 4 to 6.

Great Gazpacho (GF)

Our Gazpacho is great for warm summer evenings. Serve in place of a salad or as a first course before a Mexican meal.

4 large tomatoes (or 6 medium)

2 green onions (tops and bottoms)

3 large sprigs of parsley

1 large cucumber, peeled and seeded

2 cloves garlic, minced

2 teaspoons onion powder

1 teaspoon basil

½ teaspoon oregano

½ teaspoon thyme

2 dashes Tabasco Sauce (or ¼ teaspoon cayenne)

¼ cup apple cider vinegar

2 tablespoons concentrated apple juice

½ cup tomato puree

Puree first 10 ingredients in batches in blender or food processor. Pour mixture into a large mixing bowl. Add vinegar, apple juice and tomato puree. Chill and stir well before serving. Serves 4.

Quick Spinach-Cheese Soup

This lovely soup is very easy to prepare. Serve it with light and flavorful Banana Orange Whole Wheat Muffins and you have a delicious and nutritious meal.

1 cup Garbanzo Bean Broth, Cauliflower Broth (see chapter on Basics), or other vegetable broth
1 cup evaporated skimmed milk
1 10-ounce package frozen chopped spinach, frozen or thawed, not drained
2 teaspoons onion powder
¼ teaspoon garlic powder

1 cup low-fat cottage cheese
1 tablespoon whole wheat pastry flour

Heat first 5 ingredients in a 2-quart non-stick sauce pan over medium-high heat until mixture boils. Cover, reduce heat slightly, and cook for 7 minutes. Mix flour and cottage cheese together and stir into the soup until the cheese melts and soup thickens slightly. Do not boil. Serves 2 or 3.

Banana Orange Whole Wheat Muffins

2 large bananas, mashed (1 ¼ cups)
½ cup honey
2 tablespoons Homemade Non-Fat Yogurt or commercial brand (see chapter on Basics)
2 teaspoons cinnamon
1 teaspoon nutmeg
1 teaspoon coriander
6 egg whites
1 ½ teaspoons vanilla

2 ¼ cups whole wheat pastry flour
1 tablespoon baking soda
1 teaspoon baking powder

Continues on the next page

Whisk first 8 ingredients in a large mixing bowl. Mix together flour, soda and baking powder, and add, all at once, whisking just until blended. Fill non-stick tins ⅔ full and bake in a 350° oven for 30 minutes. Remove while still hot. Makes 18 muffins.

Creamy Cauliflower Soup (GF)

This soup is easy to make and a lovely soup to eat. Serve it with Pumpkin Raisin Muffins. The flavor and aroma of these muffins is marvelous. The dairy products in the soup And the whole grain flour- or Gluten Free flour in the muffins make this a complete and nourishing meal.

1 medium cauliflower, cut into quarters, stem removed
2 cups water
½ medium onion, cut into large chunks
3 green onions, firmly chopped
½ cup parsley leaves, chopped fine

1 cup evaporated skimmed milk
2 cups low-fat cottage cheese, whipped
⅛ to ¼ teaspoon white pepper

Cook cauliflower and vegetables in the water in a covered soup pot for 20 minutes, or until tender. Remove from heat, puree mixture, and return to pot. Stir in remaining ingredients, and heat soup slowly stirring frequently until cheese melts. Do not boil. Serves 4.

Pumpkin Raisin Muffins (or Pumpkin Raisin Bread)

2 cups canned pumpkin puree
1 ¼ cups honey
8 egg whites
1 cup evaporated skimmed milk
1 cup water
1 tablespoon oil
1 tablespoon cinnamon
1 teaspoon nutmeg
1 teaspoon ginger
¼ teaspoon cloves

3 ⅓ cups whole wheat flour
1 tablespoon baking soda

1 cup black raisins

Whisk first 10 ingredients in a large mixing bowl. Mix together flour, soda and baking powder, and add, all at once, whisking just until blended. Do not overmix. Stir in raisins. Fill non-stick muffin tins to the top and bake in a 350° oven for 30 to 35 minutes. Cool for 15 minutes before removing from pan. Batter may also be baked in two 9 ½x5 ½-inch non-stick loaf pans for 60 to 65 minutes. Yields 25 muffins.

Raisin Sweetened Whole Wheat Bran Bread

This bread contains only raisin syrup for a sweetener. It's delicious served with Homemade Apple Butter or Homemade Orange Marmalade.

1 ¼ cups bran
1 cup boiling water

Continues on the next page

4 egg whites (⅔ cup)

½ cup non-fat milk

¼ cup Non-Fat Yogurt (see chapter on Basics)

¾ cup Black Raisin Syrup (see chapter on Basics)

1 teaspoon cinnamon

1 teaspoon nutmeg

1 ½ cups whole wheat flour

1 ½ teaspoons baking soda

½ teaspoon baking powder

½ cup black raisins

Mix bran and boiling water together and set aside. Whisk the next 6 ingredients in a large mixing bowl. Mix together flour, soda and baking powder, and add, all at once, whisking just until blended. Stir in raisins and bran.

Pour batter into a 9-½x5-½-inch non-stick loaf pan, and bake in a 400° oven for 45 to 50 minutes. Allow bread to cool in a pan for at least 15 to 20 minutes. Serves 6 to 8.

Wholesome Whole Wheat Raisin-Bran Muffins

These muffins are excellent. They were inspired by sister, Joy.

2 cups bran

2 cups boiling water

2 tablespoons whole wheat pastry flour

1 cup black raisins

¾ cup honey

1 tablespoon oil

8 egg whites

1 ½ cups non-fat milk (or 2 cups buttermilk and omit yogurt)

½ cup Homemade Non-Fat Yogurt or commercial brand (see chapter on Basics)

1 ½ tablespoons cinnamon

1 tablespoon nutmeg

Continues on the next page

3 cups whole wheat pastry flour

1 tablespoon baking soda

1 teaspoon baking powder

½ cup bran

Mix together bran and boiling water and cool. Toss raisins with 2 tablespoons of flour and set aside. In a large mixing bowl whisk the next 7 ingredients. Mix together flour, baking soda and baking powder and add, all at once, whisking just until blended. Fold in bran mixture, raisin mixture and remaining ½ cup of bran. Fill non-stick muffin pans to the top and bake in a 400° oven for approximately 20 minutes. Yields 30 muffins.

Note: — Batter may be made ahead of time and stored in refrigerator for several days.

Apple Spice Bread

This bread is pure, wholesome, moist and delicious.

¾ cup frozen concentrated apple juice, unsweetened

¾ cup evaporated skimmed milk

6 egg whites

½ cup Homemade Non-Fat Yogurt or commercial brand (see chapter on Basics)

2 ½ cups whole wheat pastry flour

1 cup unprocessed bran

1 teaspoon baking powder

1 tablespoon baking soda

½ teaspoon coriander

2 teaspoons cinnamon

1 teaspoon nutmeg

½ teaspoon allspice

2 to 3 cups chopped apples, unpeeled

½ cup black raisins

½ cup chopped walnuts (optional)

Continues on the next page

Whisk first 4 ingredients in a large mixing bowl. In another bowl mix together dry ingredients and spices, and add, all at once, whisking just until blended. Stir in apples, raisins and nuts if desired. Bake in two 9x5-inch non-stick bread pans for 1 hour and 10 to 15 minutes or just until cake tester comes out clean. Do not overbake. Serves 10 to 12.

Cracked Wheat Onion Bread with Oatmeal, Bran, Chile and Cheese

Enjoy this tasty bread warm with Cottage-Chive Spread or Pimiento Spread. This bread was inspired by our niece, Elaine.

½ cup bran
1 cup cracked wheat cereal
1 cup boiling water

4 egg whites
1 cup low-fat cottage cheese
2 tablespoons non-fat yogurt
½ cup non-fat milk
⅛ teaspoon cayenne
1 tablespoon onion powder
⅛ teaspoon black pepper
2 tablespoons diced green chile peppers, canned or fresh
2 tablespoons green bell pepper
½ medium onion, chopped

1 ½ cups whole wheat flour
1 ½ teaspoons baking soda
½ teaspoon baking powder

½ cup rolled oats

Mix together cracked wheat, bran and boiling water in a small mixing bowl and set aside. Whisk next 10 ingredients in a large mixing bowl. Mix together flour, baking powder and soda, and add, all at once, whisking just until blended. Stir in oats and cereal-bran mixture.

Continues on the next page

Bake in a 400° oven in a 9 ½x5 ½-inch non-stick loaf pan for approximately 1 hour or until bread is golden brown and tests done. Let bread cool in pan for at least 15 to 20 minutes. Serves 6 to 8.

Note: — Batter may appear dry in the mixing bowl but as the bread bakes the cheese will melt and add more moisture to the loaf.

Whole Wheat Orange Raisin Yeast Muffins

¾ cup non-fat milk
¼ cup lukewarm water
1 tablespoon dry active yeast or 1 cake compressed yeast
1 tablespoon honey

5 egg whites
¼ cup honey
1 tablespoon oil
1 teaspoon cardamom
1 teaspoon cinnamon
1 teaspoon coriander
½ teaspoon Vitamin C crystals

2 cups whole wheat pastry flour

1 cup black raisins
¼ cup chopped nuts
¼ cup Cooked Orange Peel (see chapter on Basics), or 2 tablespoons grated orange peel

1 ¾ cups whole wheat pastry flour

Scald milk and cool to lukewarm. Dissolve yeast and honey in lukewarm water. In a large mixing bowl combine next 7 ingredients. Add yeast and milk and beat well with a whisk. Stir in 2 cups of flour and mix well, then add raisins, nuts and orange peel and mix again. Lastly stir in remaining flour and mix well.

Dough should be soft and will not require kneading. Cover bowl and let dough rise for 4 hours in a warm place. Knock down dough and fill non-stick muffin tins ⅔ full. Cover muffins and let dough rise again for 2 hours. Bake in a 350° oven for 35 minutes or until brown. Dough will rise as it bakes. Yields 24 muffins.

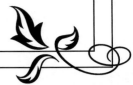

Homemade Fat-Free Banana Bread

This healthful banana bread is so good, it tastes almost like cake.

⅔ cup honey

4 egg whites

⅔ cup mashed bananas (2 small ripe bananas)

¼ cup Homemade Non-Fat Yogurt or commercial brand (see chapter on Basics)

⅓ cup non-fat milk

¼ cup evaporated skimmed milk

½ teaspoon cardamom

½ teaspoon coriander

2 ¼ cups whole wheat flour

1 teaspoon baking powder

1 tablespoon baking soda

½ cup coarsely chopped nuts or ½ cup black raisins (optional)

Whisk first 8 ingredients in a large mixing bowl. Mix together flour, baking powder and soda and add, all at once, whisking just until blended. Do not overmix. Stir in nuts or raisins. Spread batter evenly in a 9x13-inch non-stick baking pan or in two 9 ½x5 ½-inch non-stick bread pans. Bake in a 350° oven for approximately 25 to 30 minutes or just until cake tester comes out clean and bread is golden brown. Cut into squares or slices and serve warm. Serves 10 to 12.

Fat-Free and Salt-Free Corn Bread

2 egg whites
⅓ cup honey
1 ½ cups non-fat milk (or 2 cups buttermilk and omit yogurt)
½ cup Homemade Non-Fat Yogurt or commercial brand (see chapter on Basics)

1 cup cornmeal
1 cup whole wheat flour
1 teaspoon baking powder
1 teaspoon baking soda

Whisk first 4 ingredients in a large mixing bowl. Mix together cornmeal, flour, baking powder and soda and add, all at once, whisking just until smooth. Do not overbeat. Spread evenly in a 9x9-inch non-stick baking pan and bake in a 375° oven for 25 to 30 minutes or until light brown. Cut into large squares and serve warm with honey if desired. Serves 6 to 9.

SALADS & DRESSINGS

SALADS

Raw vegetable salads provide natural roughage, and are satisfying to chew. Some raw vegetables should be eaten daily. They provide many of the minerals and vitamins essential to your health. For example, leafy vegetables can give you minerals and Vitamin E; tomatoes Vitamin C; carrots and parsley Vitamin A; beets contain iron, etc.

In this section there are a variety of colorful, appealing and refreshing salads, as well as delicious tasting salad dressings, made without any salt, fat, cholesterol, or sugar.

Crunchy Cauliflower Cucumber Salad with Creamy Yogurt Dressing (GF)

This tasty crunchy salad is attractive as well as low in calories. It is also very easy to make. We use a food processor to chop and slice all the vegetables.

1 cucumber, seeded and sliced
½ medium cauliflower, broken into florets and sliced thin
¼ medium onion, chopped
1 large (or 2 small), green onion, chopped
½ small red bell pepper, chopped (or 2 tablespoons pimiento)

⅓ cup Homemade Non-Fat Yogurt or commercial brand (see chapter on Basics)
2 tablespoons cider vinegar
1 tablespoon concentrated apple juice

Place chopped and sliced vegetables in a large mixing bowl. Mix together the remaining ingredients, and stir dressing onto vegetables. Refrigerate until chilled. Serves 4 to 6.

Middle Eastern Eggplant Salad (GF)

This is the best eggplant salad we've ever tasted, and without any oil. Our friend Naomi Enoch inspired this one. It makes an excellent salad, appetizer, or buffet item.

2 medium eggplants, cut into cubes, skin left on
2 teaspoons onion powder
2 tablespoons water

1 cup celery, diced
1 cup bell pepper, diced
2 cloves garlic, minced

Continues on the next page

1 cup tomato puree

¼ teaspoon cayenne

1 tablespoon cumin

2 tablespoons concentrated apple juice

¼ cup wine vinegar

1 tablespoon parsley, chopped

Cook eggplant cubes and onion powder covered in non-stick frying pan with 2 tablespoons of water, for approximately 10 to 15 minutes, or until eggplant is tender. Place eggplant into a mixing bowl. In the same pan stir-fry celery, bell pepper and garlic until tender, for approximately 10 minutes, then return eggplant to frying pan. Stir in next 5 ingredients and cook, uncovered, for 20 minutes. Stir in parsley and refrigerate. Serves 6 to 8.

Quick Tomato Salad Dressing (GF)

This tasty dressing can be made quickly in the blender or food processor.

2 medium tomatoes, chopped fine

2 tablespoons lemon juice

1 tablespoon wine vinegar

⅛ teaspoon ground pepper

2 tablespoons minced green onion

2 tablespoons minced parsley

1 tablespoon fresh herbs, minced, (or 1 teaspoon dried herbs, crumbled)

Puree all ingredients in a blender or food processor, and refrigerate until serving. Yields 1 cup of dressing.

Marinated Garbanzo Beans with Flo's French Herb Dressing (GF)

Garbanzo beans are an excellent source of protein, and they taste marvelous marinated in this herb dressing. Use this dressing also for mixed green salads, or spoon it over sliced tomatoes. It's great tasting, and without any oil or salt.

3 cups cooked garbanzo beans
½ cup Flo's French Herb Dressing

Toss garbanzo beans with dressing and allow beans to marinate for several hours or preferably overnight. Serves 4 to 6.

Flo's French Herb Dressing (GF)

1 cup red wine vinegar
½ teaspoon ground pepper
2 cloves crushed garlic
1 teaspoon dried mustard
½ teaspoon tarragon
½ teaspoon oregano
1 teaspoon basil
1 teaspoon dried dill weed
½ teaspoon rosemary
1 teaspoon paprika
1 tablespoon honey
1 tablespoon lemon juice
½ cup chopped parsley
1 teaspoon onion powder

Mix all ingredients together well, and store dressing in refrigerator. Yields 1 ¼ cups of dressing.

Winter Fresh Fruit Salad with Lemon Yogurt Dressing (GF)

Enjoy winter and summer fruits with Lemon Yogurt Dressing. We also spoon this delicious dressing over cottage cheese and fruit any time of the year.

3 oranges, peeled
3 sweet apples, unpeeled, cored, and cut into quarters
3 large bananas

Cut fruit into bite-sized pieces and chill. Serve fruit salad in small dessert bowls, and pass the Lemon Yogurt Dressing. Serves 3 to 4.

Lemon Yogurt Dressing (GF)

1 cup Homemade Non-Fat Yogurt or commercial brand (see chapter on Basics)
2 tablespoons fresh lemon juice
1 tablespoon honey

Mix ingredients together and chill. Makes 1 cup of dressing.

Marinated Bean Salad with Pimiento (GF)

This attractive and tasty bean salad provides added protein to a vegetarian meal. It makes an excellent salad for a buffet.

2 cups cooked garbanzo beans, drained
2 packages frozen cut green beans, cooked just until tender and drained
1 cucumber, sliced thin

Continues on the next page

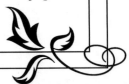

1 teaspoon dried dill weed

1 teaspoon dried oregano, crumbled

⅛ teaspoon ground pepper

1 4-ounce jar diced pimientos

¼ cup wine vinegar

2 tablespoons lemon juice

1 teaspoon onion powder

Mix together all ingredients well and refrigerate for at least 2 hours. Serves 4 to 6.

Red Cabbage Slaw (GF)

This attractive, easy-to-prepare slaw is best made the day before.

½ cup cider vinegar

2 tablespoons concentrated apple juice

2 tablespoons water

½ teaspoon ground ginger

¼ teaspoon pepper (white or black)

1 medium head of red cabbage, shredded by hand, or in food processor, using slicer attachment

½ cup parsley leaves, chopped

Bring first 5 ingredients to a boil in a small saucepan over medium heat. Cook dressing for 3 minutes. Place shredded cabbage in a large mixing bowl and pour hot dressing over cabbage. Stir in parsley and toss well. Refrigerate until serving. Serves 6 to 8.

Pineapple Cole Slaw (GF)

4 cups shredded cabbage
1 red bell pepper (or green, if red is not available), chopped
½ cup white vinegar
½ cup unsweetened pineapple juice
1 tablespoon honey
½ cup crushed pineapple or chunks

Mix together all ingredients well, and chill in refrigerator until serving. Serves 4 to 6.

Rice Vinegar Mustard Dressing (GF)

Use this light flavorful dressing over mixed greens, with tomato wedges and cucumbers.

1 cup rice vinegar (rice vinegar is quite mild)
½ teaspoon black pepper
2 tablespoons lemon juice
2 tablespoons honey
2 tablespoons salt-free mustard
3 cloves garlic
3 green onions, cut into quarters lengthwise

Mix together all ingredients in blender, and store dressing in refrigerator. Yields 1 ½ cups of dressing.

Non-Fat Green Yogurt Dressing (GF)

This is a very tasty and thick dressing.

⅔ cup Non-Fat Yogurt (see chapter on Basics)
1 cup parsley leaves
6 green onions
3 tablespoons apple cider vinegar
3 tablespoons lemon juice
2 tablespoons concentrated frozen apple juice
¼ teaspoon black pepper

Mix together all the ingredients in a blender or food processor, and chill before serving. Yields 1 ½ cups of dressing.

Tangy Salad Dressing (GF)

Use this tangy dressing on salads or with any raw vegetables.

¼ cup wine vinegar
1 tablespoon fresh lemon juice
2 tablespoons Homemade Salt-Free Chili Sauce, (see chapter on Condiments)
⅛ teaspoon black pepper

Mix all ingredients together well, and refrigerate. Yields ½ cup of dressing.

Yogurt-Sesame Seed Dressing (GF)

This excellent dressing tastes best a few days after it is made. It is one of our favorites.

1 cup Non-Fat Yogurt, (see chapter on Basics)
¼ cup hulled sesame seeds
1 clove garlic
½ tablespoon fresh parsley
½ teaspoon dried dill weed
1 tablespoon lemon juice
1 tablespoon red wine vinegar

Mix together all ingredients well in a blender or food processor, and refrigerate. Yields 1 ½ cups of dressing.

Marinated Vegetable Salad with Easy Vinaigrette Dressing (GF)

Enjoy this crunchy salad with this light, tasty vinaigrette dressing.

4 carrots, sliced
4 stalks of celery, sliced
½ medium bell pepper, cut in strips, or sliced
2 zucchini, sliced
2 cups cauliflower pieces or sliced

Toss sliced vegetables in dressing, and allow to marinate for several hours, or preferably overnight. Serves 4 to 6.

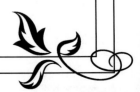

Easy Vinaigrette Dressing (GF)

2 tablespoons Dijon mustard
¼ cup red wine vinegar
¼ teaspoon ground pepper
2 tablespoons lemon juice

Whisk mustard, vinegar, lemon juice and pepper in small bowl until blended and refrigerate. Yields ¾ cup of dressing.

Tofu Jalapeno Salad (GF)

This is an excellent, spicy, non-dairy salad. It makes a colorful and unusual buffet dish too.

1 recipe Scrambled Tofu Jalapeno (see Index)

3 fresh tomatoes, chopped
1 bell pepper, chopped
¼ small onion, chopped

Allow scrambled tofu to cool. Stir in raw vegetables, and chill salad in refrigerator until ready to serve. Serves 4 to 6.

Marinated Cucumber Salad (GF)

This tangy, crispy salad is easy to prepare and makes a fine salad for buffets.

3 medium cucumbers

1 large green onion

¼ cup fresh parsley leaves

1 tablespoon concentrated apple juice
⅓ cup white vinegar
½ teaspoon celery seed
¼ teaspoon black pepper
2 teaspoons onion powder

Peel and thinly slice cucumbers by hand or in food processor. Chop green onion and parsley. Mix together all ingredients in a large mixing bowl, and marinate salad in refrigerator for at least 6 hours or overnight. Serves 4 to 6.

Marinated Tangy Beet Salad (GF)

This lovely tasting salad is colorful for a buffet and complements any meal.

1 large bunch beets, peeled

3 tablespoons red wine vinegar
3 tablespoons beet broth (from cooking the beets)
1 tablespoon concentrated apple juice
¼ teaspoon powdered horseradish
1 teaspoon onion powder
1 teaspoon ground coriander
⅛ teaspoon black pepper

Continues on the next page

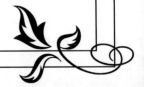

Cook beets until tender in enough water to cover. Young beets take approximately 45 minutes to cook. Older beets take from 1 ½ to 2 hours. Reserve part of beet broth for marinade. Cut cooked beets in small cubes, or julienne, by hand or in a food processor.

Mix together all ingredients for the marinade in a medium-sized mixing bowl and toss well. Allow beets to marinate for several hours or preferably overnight. Serves 4 to 6.

Carrot-Raisin-Celery Salad with Orange Yogurt Dressing (GF)

This delicious salad is healthy and attractive. The Orange Yogurt Dressing beautifully enhances the flavors of the vegetables.

6 cups of grated carrots
1 cup raisins
2 cups sliced celery
¼ cup walnut chunks (optional)

Mix salad ingredients together and toss well with enough dressing to moisten. Refrigerate. Serves 4 to 6.

Orange Yogurt Dressing (GF)

¼ cup concentrated frozen orange juice
½ cup Homemade Non-Fat Yogurt or commercial brand (see chapter on Basics)
½ teaspoon coriander

Mix together and chill. Makes ¾ cup of dressing.

Cucumber Salad with Pimientos (GF)

This is a refreshing, low-calorie salad. Buy thin young cucumbers with small seeds if possible.

4 medium cucumbers, sliced thin
¼ cup white vinegar
1 tablespoon honey
2 tablespoons diced green pepper
1 2-ounce jar of diced pimiento

Mix together all ingredients. Toss, and chill for several hours. Serves 4 to 6.

MAIN COURSES

Main Courses

What a pleasure it is to prepare and serve a wide variety of delicious, nourishing and satisfying entrees, made with little or no fat, cholesterol or salt.

In this section you will find marvelous recipes for vegetarian entrees, casseroles, crepes, quiches, souffles, omelettes, vegi loaves and burgers, pasta dishes, and Italian, French, Greek, Jewish, American, Oriental and Mexican specialties, as well as spectacular holiday and party entrees. You will be able to serve dishes that will truly please your palate and satisfy your body; and you will be getting the nutrients, vitamins and minerals that your body needs to feel energetic, strong and satisfied.

Whole Wheat Spinach or Gluten free Noodles with Salsa Fresca (GF)

(Italian Tomato Sauce)

Isolina Ricci, an Italian friend of mine, inspired this one. The longer you cook the sauce the sweeter the onion and garlic become. You can also serve this sauce over brown rice.

1 large onion, chopped
3 large cloves garlic, minced

2 teaspoons oregano
2 teaspoons basil
1 teaspoon thyme

6 medium tomatoes (or 8 smaller ones), chopped
1 cup tomato puree

1 pound whole wheat spinach noodles

Brown onion and garlic in a non-stick saucepan. As onion begins to brown, stir in a few drops of water to moisten, and continue browning. When moisture is gone stir in herbs, then add chopped tomatoes and tomato puree. Simmer sauce uncovered for 1 hour or longer if possible.

Ten minutes before serving, cook noodles until tender, drain and rinse, in hot water. Serve with sauce. Serves 6.

Superb Spinach-Cheese Lasagna (GF)

This superb lasagna is a great party dish. It can be prepared the day before and stored in refrigerator until 1 hour before baking. This is one of our family favorites. Serve with big tossed salad and Minestrone Soup.

Continues on the next page

Sauce:
1 large onion, chopped
6 cloves garlic, minced

4 cups tomato puree
1 teaspoon onion powder
1 tablespoon Italian seasonings
¼ teaspoon black pepper

Saute the onion and garlic in a non-stick frying pan, adding a little water several times as needed to keep onions from sticking and burning. When onions are soft add tomato puree, onion powder, and seasonings. Simmer sauce slowly for 25 minutes and remove from heat.

Pasta:
1 pound whole wheat or Gluten free lasagna noodles, cooked until tender

While sauce is cooking heat water for lasagna noodles in a large pot until water is boiling rapidly. Add noodles, and cook according to instructions on package. Rinse and leave the noodles in cool water until ready to use. Drain noodles well just before assembling lasagna.

Cheese-Spinach Filling:
4 cups low-fat cottage cheese, whipped
2 teaspoons onion powder
½ teaspoon garlic powder

2 packages frozen chopped spinach (10 ounces each package), thawed

Mix together whipped cottage cheese, onion and garlic powder and set aside. Squeeze out spinach and set aside.

To assemble: Layer lasagna in a 9x13-inch non-stick or glass oven-proof baking pan in the following order: (1) 1 cup of sauce for bottom of pan, (2) a layer of noodles, (3) ¾ cup sauce spread over noodles, (4) ½ of cottage cheese over noodles, (5) ½ of spinach on top of cottage cheese, (6) another layer of noodles, (7) repeat #3, 4, 5, and 6, (8) top with sauce. Bake lasagna in a 350° oven for 1 hour or until hot and bubbly, and light brown on top. Let stand for a few minutes before serving. Serves 6 to 8.

Magnificent Manicotti Marinara Casserole

This is an elegant party entree that can be prepared the day before and stored in refrigerator until 1 hour before baking time. The taste and aroma is divine. A huge vegetable salad tossed with Flo's French Herb Dressing goes perfectly with this.

24 7-inch Tender Whole Wheat Crepes (see chapter on Basics)

Marinara Sauce:
1 large onion, chopped
6 cloves garlic, minced
¼ teaspoon pepper
1 teaspoon basil
1 teaspoon oregano
1 tablespoon fresh parsley, minced (or 1 teaspoon dried parsley)

1 can #2 ½ tomato puree (3 ½ cups)
1 teaspoon apple cider vinegar
¼ cup water

Saute the onion, garlic and herbs in a non-stick frying pan until brown, adding 1 or 2 tablespoons of water as needed. Stir in tomato puree, vinegar and water. Simmer covered over low heat for 30 minutes, stirring occasionally.

Cheese Filling:
6 cups (3 pounds) low-fat cottage cheese, whipped
2 tablespoons potato starch or cornstarch
2 tablespoons whole wheat pastry flour
2 tablespoons finely chopped parsley
1 ½ teaspoons dried sweet basil, crushed
¼ teaspoon ground pepper
1 tablespoon onion powder
1 teaspoon garlic powder

While the sauce is cooking whisk all the cheese filling ingredients in a large mixing bowl.

Continues on the next page

To assemble Manicotti Casserole: Spoon a thin layer of sauce on the bottom of two 9x13-inch non-stick baking pans. Place a generous amount of cheese mixture in the center of each crepe and roll up. Arrange manicotti in both pans. Cover with sauce. Bake in a 400° oven for approximately 30 to 35 minutes or just until puffed and bubbly. Do not overbake. Allow to set for 5 minutes before serving. Serves 8 to 10.

Eggplant Parmigiana with Tomato Mushroom Sauce

This is a lovely entree to serve. Most eggplant parmigiana is prepared with a lot of oil and cheese. Ours, made with homemade Tomato Mushroom Sauce, has all the goodness and very little cholesterol, salt or fat.

2 medium eggplants, cut into ½-inch slices, skin left on

1 cup Tomato Mushroom Sauce (or more as desired)

2 cups low-fat cottage cheese
1 tablespoon whole wheat pastry flour
1 teaspoon onion powder
½ teaspoon garlic powder

6 medium mushrooms, sliced
1 teaspoon Italian seasonings, crushed for top

Soak eggplant slices in water for 10 to 15 minutes and drain. Fry slices on a hot, non-stick griddle without oil until brown on both sides and until barely tender when pierced with a fork. Remove from heat.

Preheat oven to 350°. Place 2 tablespoons of the sauce on the bottom of a 9x13-inch non-stick or glass oven-proof baking dish. Arrange half the eggplant slices on top of sauce and spread a tablespoon of sauce on top of each eggplant slice.

Blend the cottage cheese, flour, and seasonings in a blender or food processor. Spread cottage cheese mixture over eggplant slices. Place remaining eggplant slices on top, and cover with remaining sauce. Top with Italian seasonings and mushrooms and bake in a 350° oven for 30 minutes or until bubbly and heated through. Let stand for 5 minutes before serving. Serves 6.

Tomato Mushroom Sauce (GF)

1 medium onion, minced
2 cloves garlic, minced
2 tablespoons water

2 cups tomato puree

¼ cup minced parsley
2 teaspoons dried Italian seasonings (herbs), crumbled (or 2 tablespoons minced fresh
    herbs)
dash pepper
½ pound mushrooms, sliced

In a non-stick saucepan, saute onion, garlic, and water until softened. Add tomato puree and simmer slowly for approximately 15 minutes until moisture is reduced, stirring frequently to prevent burning. Stir in remaining ingredients and simmer for 5 minutes longer.

Mountain of Crepes a la Florentine

This healthy, delicious, exciting and impressive entree is sure to bring oohs and aahs. It can be prepared entirely the day or evening before. Remove from refrigerator 2 hours before heating.

24 7-inch Tender Whole Wheat Crepes (see chapter on Basics)

Spinach Filling for Crepes:
1 ½ medium onions, chopped
9 cloves garlic, minced
1 ½ medium green bell peppers, chopped
½ cup parsley leaves, chopped
2 tablespoons dried sweet basil
½ teaspoon black pepper
¼ teaspoon nutmeg

Continues on the next page

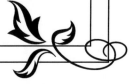

3 10-ounce packages frozen chopped spinach, thawed and drained, not squeezed out

1 ½ cups evaporated skimmed milk

3 cups low-fat cottage cheese

Saute first 7 ingredients in a large non-stick frying pan. When pan becomes dry add thawed spinach. Cook over medium heat until most of the moisture is gone. Stir in milk to cool mixture down, then stir in cottage cheese and cook until cheese begins to melt. Do not allow mixture to boil once cheese has been added. Remove from heat and set aside.

Cheese Sauce:
½ pound mushrooms, chopped fine
1 large onion, chopped fine
4 garlic cloves

5 tablespoons whole wheat pastry flour
1 cup evaporated skimmed milk
1 cup non-fat milk
1 tablespoon onion powder
½ teaspoon ground pepper
¼ teaspoon nutmeg
2 teaspoons thyme
1 teaspoon basil
dash cinnamon

3 cups low-fat cottage cheese

In a large non-stick saucepan saute mushrooms, onions and garlic until moisture is absorbed. Stir in next 9 ingredients. Stir the sauce over low heat until it comes to a boil. Allow sauce to boil for 1 minute stirring constantly. Stir in cottage cheese until sauce is hot again, and cheese begins to melt. Remove from heat before sauce comes to a boil. Set sauce aside.

To assemble Mountain Of Crepes: Pour ¼ cup of the cheese sauce into a 2-quart souffle dish. Stack crepes in the souffle dish with 1 heaping tablespoon of spinach filling between each crepe layer. Pour enough sauce over Mountain Of Crepes to cover top and sides well. Reserve additional sauce in a saucepan, and heat just before serving to spoon over each portion.

Bake Mountain Of Crepes in a 375° oven for approximately 1 hour, or until crepes and filling are heated through, and the top is light brown and bubbly. Cut into wedges and spoon cheese sauce on top. Serves 6 to 8.

Fabulous Low-Fat Fettucine Alfredo (GF)

Fettucine Alfredo is an exciting and elegant dish to serve. You can eat all you want of ours. Most of the fat and cholesterol are left out, but the flavor is left in.

½ pound mushrooms, sliced

6 cloves garlic, minced

2 cups chopped onions

2 teaspoons Italian seasonings, crumbled

1 teaspoon dried basil crumbled

¼ cup white wine (optional)

¾ cup evaporated skimmed milk

¾ cup water

2 tablespoons whole wheat flour or Gluten Free flour

2 teaspoons onion powder

¼ teaspoon white pepper

3 cups low-fat cottage cheese

¼ cup chopped parsley

1 tablespoon garlic powder

⅛ teaspoon nutmeg

1 pound whole wheat or Gluten free fettucine or linguine, cooked tender but firm and
    drained

Saute first 6 ingredients in a large frying pan until moisture is absorbed. Set aside. In a small non-stick saucepan bring the next 5 sauce ingredients to a boil and cook for 5 minutes, stirring frequently. Stir sauce into sauteed mushroom mixture, along with cottage cheese, and heat just until cottage cheese melts. Do not boil sauce. Toss pasta and sauce together in frying pan or large pot, and heat for 5 minutes. During the last 30 seconds stir in the chopped parsley, garlic powder and nutmeg, and serve at once. Serves 8.

Fettucine Primavera (GF)

This combination of whole wheat pasta, vegetables and creamy cheese sauce makes a delicious, wholesome meal, that is seasoned just right.

2 cups chopped broccoli, fresh or frozen
2 cups chopped cauliflower, fresh or frozen
1 cup chopped onion
1 tablespoon Italian seasonings, crumbled

¾ cup evaporated skimmed milk
¾ cup water
2 tablespoons whole wheat flour or Gluten Free flour
1 tablespoon onion powder
¼ teaspoon black pepper

3 cups low-fat cottage cheese

1 pound whole wheat or Gluten free fettucine or broad noodles, cooked tender but firm and drained

2 green onions, chopped
¼ cup chopped fresh parsley
1 tablespoon garlic powder
1 tablespoon lemon juice
½ teaspoon coriander

Saute vegetables and Italian seasonings in a large non-stick frying pan until moisture is absorbed. Set aside. Bring next 5 sauce ingredients to a boil in a small non-stick saucepan, and cook for 5 minutes, stirring frequently. Stir sauce into sauteed vegetable mixture along with cottage cheese, and heat just until cottage cheese melts. Do not boil sauce. Toss pasta and sauce together in frying pan or large pot, and heat for 5 minutes. During the last 30 seconds stir in remaining ingredients and serve at once. Serves 8.

Cheesy Whole Wheat or Gluten free Shells with Flavorful Bell Pepper-Tomato Sauce (GF)

Whole wheat shells taste delicious all coated with cheese sauce and topped with Flavorful Bell Pepper-Tomato Sauce. A fresh green salad will complete this healthy, well balanced meal.

1 pound large or medium whole wheat shells

2 cups low-fat cottage cheese
1 tablespoon non-fat milk
1 tablespoon onion powder
2 teaspoons Italian seasonings
¼ cup chopped parsley
¼ teaspoon ground pepper
1 teaspoon garlic powder

Heat water for pasta in a large pot. Cook shells until tender, rinse and drain well in cold water. Meanwhile prepare cheese sauce by heating the remaining ingredients in a large frying pan, just until the cheese begins to melt. Remove from heat until pasta is ready. Over low heat stir shells in cheese sauce until all shells are coated and hot. Spoon Flavorful Bell Pepper-Tomato Sauce over each serving. Serves 6.

Flavorful Bell Pepper-Tomato Sauce (GF)

1 medium onion
5 cloves of garlic
1 large green bell pepper
1 tablespoon Italian seasonings

3 cups tomato puree
¼ cup water

Chop the vegetables and Italian seasonings in a food processor or blender, or by hand. Saute this mixture until vegetables are slightly browned. Stir in tomato puree and water, and simmer for 20 to 30 minutes. Yields 1-quart of sauce.

Baked Mushroom Egg White Omelette
with Spicy Spanish Sauce

Serve this delicious omelette topped with Spicy Spanish Sauce.

½ medium onion, chopped
½ small green bell pepper, chopped
¼ small red bell pepper, chopped (or 2 tablespoons chopped pimiento)
2 large (or 3 small), green onions, chopped
½ pound mushrooms, sliced
1 teaspoon Italian seasonings, crumbled
⅛ teaspoon black pepper

1 cup low-fat cottage cheese
2 tablespoons whole wheat pastry flour
1 tablespoon onion powder
⅛ teaspoon turmeric
1 teaspoon sweet basil
1 teaspoon thyme

12 egg whites
½ teaspoon potato starch or cornstarch
sprinkle of crumbled oregano for top

Saute first 7 ingredients in a non-stick frying pan for 7 minutes and set aside. Mix together cottage cheese, flour, onion powder and seasonings in a small bowl and set aside. Beat egg whites and starch in an electric mixer until whites are stiff but not dry. Lightly fold in cottage cheese-flour mixture and sauteed vegetables while beating on low speed.

Spread mixture into a 9x9-inch non-stick baking pan. Sprinkle with oregano and bake in a 325° oven for approximately 25 minutes or until knife comes out clean. Cut generous slices and top with sauce. Serves 3 or 4.

Spicy Spanish Sauce:
½ medium onion, minced
½ medium green bell pepper, chopped

Continues on the next page

2 cups tomato puree

½ teaspoon chili powder

1 teaspoon cider vinegar or red wine vinegar

Saute onion and bell pepper in a non-stick frying pan for 5 minutes. Stir in tomato puree, chili powder and vinegar. Simmer sauce for 15 minutes and serve over baked omelette. Yields 2 cups of sauce.

Vegi Chili Beans with Spanish Rice (GF)

This substantial, tasty Mexican meal can serve a big family for pennies. The spicy beans and tasty Spanish Rice combine to make a well-balanced protein-carbohydrate meal to boost your energy.

3 cups dried kidney, or small red beans

water to cover well

3 medium onions (3 cups), chopped

3 large cloves of garlic, minced

1 green bell pepper

1 teaspoon onion powder

1 teaspoon garlic powder

1 tablespoon cumin

1 teaspoon oregano

1 tablespoon chili powder

2 cups tomato puree

3 ½ cups hot water

2 tablespoons cider vinegar

4 green onions, chopped, for garnish

Bring beans and water to a boil in a large pot (covered), and boil vigorously for 10 minutes. Allow beans to remain in hot water until cool or overnight. Discard liquid, rinse beans and return beans to pot, or to a large crockpot.

Continues on the next page

Saute the onions, garlic, and bell pepper in a non-stick frying pan, adding a little water as needed. Stir in spices and seasonings, and continue frying until onions and bell pepper are softened and moisture is absorbed.

Stir 3 ½ cups hot water, tomato puree and sauteed vegetables into pot with beans.

To cook beans on top of stove: Bring beans to boil, cover, and cook very slowly. Stir beans occasionally, so that they do not stick and burn. Cook until beans are tender, for approximately 2 ½ to 3 hours.

To cook in crockpot: Cook beans for 8 to 10 hours before mealtime. Set crockpot temperature gauge on high temperature and go to work or about your daily routine until mealtime.

Ten minutes before serving add vinegar. Sprinkle green onions on top of each serving. Serves 8 to 10.

Note: — In case the Vegi Chili is too thin, cook it uncovered, stirring occasionally, for 20 to 30 minutes, or until beans are the desired consistency.

Spanish Rice (GF)

1 onion, diced
1 red or green bell pepper, diced
2 cloves garlic, minced

6 ripe tomatoes, cut into pieces

2 ½ cups brown rice, raw
4 cups boiling water

Saute onion, bell pepper and garlic, uncovered, until brown, in a large non-stick frying pan that has a tight fitting lid. Add small amounts of water to keep vegetables from sticking, then mix in tomatoes and bring to a boil. Stir in rice and boiling water and cover pan. Lower heat and cook until water is absorbed for approximately 40 minutes. Serves 8 to 10.

Baked Potatoes Stuffed with Cheese and Green Onions (GF)

These deliciously warming, stuffed baked potatoes can be frozen before or after baking. When served with a salad and cooked vegetables, this potato-cheese combination provides a nutritious protein entree.

6 medium-sized potatoes, baked until soft

2 cups low-fat cottage cheese
2 teaspoons onion powder
¼ teaspoon ground pepper
2 to 4 tablespoons evaporated skimmed milk or non-fat milk

6 green onions, top and white parts, chopped

sprinkle of paprika

Cut potatoes in half lengthwise. Scoop out insides and reserve outer skins intact. Puree potatoes with cottage cheese, onion powder, pepper and enough milk to allow food processor or blender blades to move. Stir in green onions and fill potato skins; arrange potato halves in a 10x15-inch non-stick jelly roll pan. Sprinkle paprika on top and bake in a 450° oven for 20 to 30 minutes until very light brown on top and just heated through. Serves 8 to 10.

Note: – *Potatoes can be baked the day before and refrigerated, but it is easier to scoop out potatoes when they are still warm. Before heating stuffed potatoes have them stay out of refrigerator for 1 hour.*

Nachos Supreme with Cooked Chili Salsa (GF)

This is especially fun to eat. The combination of ingredients are well-balanced to give you the protein and complex carbohydrates you need for a healthy body. You can serve this for an entree or appetizer with Cooked Chili Salsa Sauce spooned on top, and a dollop of Mock Sour Cream.

Continues on the next page

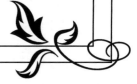

1 tablespoon onion powder

1 tablespoon chili powder

¼ cup warm water

12 corn tortillas (made without lard and preservatives)

2 cups Spicy Refried Beans (see chapter on Basics)

1 cup chopped onions

Mix together onion powder, chili powder and water in cup. Take 1 teaspoonful of this mixture and spread it over one side of each tortilla. Cut tortillas in eighths and bake in a 400° oven in a 10x15-inch non-stick jelly roll pan for approximately 10 minutes on each side, or until crispy on both sides.

To assemble: Place tortilla chips in a 9-inch glass oven-proof pie plate. Spoon hot refried beans on top of chips. Spoon heated Cooked Chili Salsa Sauce over beans and sprinkle onions on top. Place under broiler for a few minutes until very hot. Serve at once. Serves 4.

Cooked Chili Salsa (GF)

2 cups chopped tomatoes

½ cup chopped onions

¼ cup chopped chile peppers (or 1 4-ounce can diced green chiles)

⅛ teaspoon ground pepper

2 tablespoons white vinegar

Simmer all ingredients in a saucepan for 15 minutes. Store in refrigerator and use sparingly on Nachos Supreme and other Mexican dishes. Yields 2 cups of salsa.

Fast Taco Salad with Mild Chile Salsa (GF)

This cold salad, with hot beans and mild salsa makes a satisfying meal in minutes. Top with a dollop of Mock Sour Cream if desired.

½ medium head of iceberg, or Romaine lettuce, shredded fine
3 or 4 medium tomatoes, chopped
1 cucumber (seeded if seeds are large), chopped
1 green or red bell pepper, chopped
¼ small onion, finely chopped

2 cups Spicy Refried Beans or Vegi Chili Beans (see chapter on Basics)

Prepare vegetables and chill. Before serving heat beans. Pile salad on 2 large dinner plates. Spoon a mound of hot beans in the center of each salad. Top with the Mild Chile Salsa, or Hot Salsa (see Index). Serve at once. Serves 2.

Mild Chile Salsa (GF)

1 cup chopped tomatoes
¼ cup chopped onions
1 tablespoon chopped fresh or canned diced chile pepper
dash ground pepper
1 tablespoon white vinegar

Simmer all ingredients in a saucepan for 10 to 15 minutes. Store in refrigerator. Yields 1 ⅓ cups of salsa.

Easy Spicy Mexican Rice-Cheese Bake (GF)

Easy to fix, fun to eat and healthy for you! Serve with a big salad.

4 cups low-fat cottage cheese, whipped
½ cup chopped fresh green chile peppers (or 2 4-ounce cans diced green chile peppers)
2 teaspoons onion powder

4 cups cooked brown rice (2 cups raw brown rice cooked in 4 cups water with 2
    teaspoons onion powder added)
2 cups frozen or fresh corn kernels

Mix together cottage cheese, onion powder and chiles. Stir in rice and corn. Spread in a 9x13-inch non-stick or glass oven-proof baking dish and bake in a 325° oven for 30 to 35 minutes, or until casserole is heated through. Serves 6.

Vegetarian Low-Fat Mexican Corn and Cheese Casserole (GF)

At last—great low-fat Mexican food without lard. We appreciate it especially because we can't find it anywhere else. Now you can enjoy it too. Serve with a raw vegetable salad.

1 quart Home-Made Enchilada Sauce (see chapter on Basics)

18 corn tortillas

3 cups low-fat cottage cheese
2 teaspoons onion powder
½ teaspoon garlic powder

2 cups frozen or fresh corn kernels

2 tablespoons chopped fresh green chile peppers (or 2-ounces canned diced green chile
    peppers, or more if desired)

½ medium onion chopped for topping

To assemble casserole: Reserve 1 ½ cups of enchilada sauce to heat before serving. Pour ½ cup enchilada sauce in the bottom of a 9x13-inch non-stick baking pan and arrange 6 tortillas on top of the sauce. Pour ¾ cup sauce over tortillas. Mix together cottage cheese, onion powder and garlic powder, and spread 1 ½ cups of cottage cheese mixture over tortillas. Sprinkle 1 cup corn kernels over cottage cheese, and 1-ounce of the chile peppers. Repeat all these layers once again.

To complete the casserole arrange the 6 remaining tortillas on top. Pour 1 cup of sauce over top, and sprinkle with chopped onions. Bake casserole in 350° oven for approximately 45 minutes to 1 hour, or until casserole is very hot and bubbly. Serve with heated enchilada sauce spooned over serving. Serves 8.

Mexican Tostadas (GF)

Tostados are an exciting treat! Serve with Hot Salsa, used very sparingly.

½ cup chopped onion
4 tomatoes, diced
1 medium green bell pepper, diced
2 cups shredded lettuce

2 cups Spicy Refried Beans (see chapter on Basics)

1 cup Home-Made Enchilada Sauce (see chapter on Basics)

4 corn tortillas

Toss together salad vegetables in a bowl, and chill before serving. Heat beans and sauce separately. Toast tortillas lightly in toaster oven, or on a cookie sheet in the oven.

To assemble tostada: Place 1 toasted tortilla on each dinner plate. Spread ½ cup of beans on top of each toasted tortilla, ¼ cup of sauce on top of beans, one-fourth of the salad vegetables on each, a bit of hot salsa, and a dollop of Mock Sour Cream or Creamy Cottage Cheese, if you like. Serves 3 to 4.

Note: – The beans and sauce can be made a day or two beforehand. The salad can be made in the morning before serving.

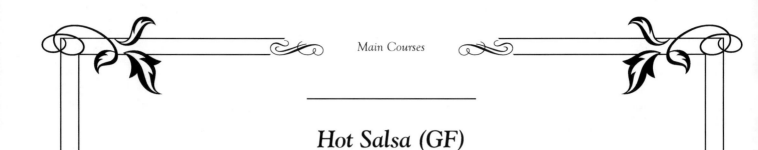
Hot Salsa (GF)

3 or 4 ripe tomatoes (1 pound), diced

¼ cup chopped fresh green chile peppers (or 1 4-ounce can diced green chiles)
2 tablespoons vinegar
1 jalapeno pepper, chopped
6 green onions, chopped

Cook tomatoes for 15 minutes uncovered. Cool. Mix in remaining ingredients. Refrigerate for at least 24 hours before serving.

Tasty Tamale Pie Casserole (GF)

This zesty tamale pie is exciting to eat. We enjoy it topped with a dollop of Mock Sour Cream, or Creamy Whipped Cottage Cheese, and a big salad. What could be better?

2 cups Home-Made Enchilada Sauce (see chapter on Basics)

2 cups cornmeal
5 ½ cups water
2 teaspoons chili powder
4 teaspoons onion powder

1 ½ cups low-fat cottage cheese

2 cups frozen or fresh corn kernels

1 recipe Spicy Refried Beans (see chapter on Basics)

½ cup chopped onions

Reserve ¾ cup of enchilada sauce to heat before serving. Mix together cornmeal, water and spices into a large saucepan. Stir frequently as mixture thickens. Remove from heat.

Continues on the next page

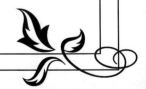

To assemble tamale pie: Pour ¼ cup of enchilada sauce into the bottom of a 9x13-inch non-stick or glass oven-proof baking pan. Spread cornmeal on bottom and along sides of baking dish. Pour ½ cup of sauce over cornmeal, then spread cottage cheese over cornmeal, sprinkle corn kernels over cottage cheese, then spread beans over the corn kernels. Pour ½ cup of sauce over beans and sprinkle chopped onions on top. Bake in a 350° oven for 45 minutes. Heat ¾ cup of sauce to spoon over top of each portion. Serves 3 to 4.

Vegetarian Low-Fat Mexican Casserole (GF)

This easy-to-prepare, exciting casserole is the perfect dish to bring to a potluck supper, or to serve at your own parties. It can be prepared a day ahead of time and even frozen. This combination of ingredients provides a completely healthy balanced meal. Serve casserole with salad, chopped onions, and Whipped Cottage Cheese Topping.

1 quart Home-Made Enchilada Sauce (see chapter on Basics)

18 corn tortillas

3 cups Spicy Refried Beans (see chapter on Basics)

2 cups (1 pound) low-fat cottage cheese
1 teaspoon onion powder
½ teaspoon garlic powder

1 10-ounce package frozen corn kernels
2 tablespoons chopped fresh green chile peppers, or 2 ounces canned diced green chile peppers

Reserve 1 ⅓ cups of Enchilada Sauce to heat before serving. Layer a 9x13-inch non-stick baking pan as follows: Pour ⅔ cup sauce into bottom of pan. Arrange 6 tortillas on top of sauce, pour beans on top of tortillas, cover beans with 6 more tortillas, and pour 1 cup sauce over tortillas. Mix together onion and garlic powder with cottage cheese and place large spoonfuls of cheese mixture evenly on top of tortillas. Sprinkle corn and chile peppers on top of cottage cheese, arrange last 6 tortillas on top, and pour 1 cup of sauce over tortillas.

Bake casserole in a 350° oven uncovered for 1 hour or until casserole is very hot and bubbly.

Before serving heat reserved sauce in a saucepan, and spoon sauce over each portion. Serves 8 to 10.

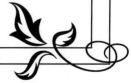

Cheese-Onion Souffle with Fresh Herbs and Crockpot Carrot-Sweet Potato Tzimmes

Can you imagine how good it will feel to serve this beautiful and flavorful souffle, and know that it is good for you and your loved ones. For an extra treat serve this souffle with Carrot-Sweet Potato Tzimmes which can be prepared ahead of time.

3 cups low-fat cottage cheese
1 tablespoon onion powder
1 teaspoon garlic powder
¼ teaspoon black pepper
3 tablespoons whole wheat pastry flour
3 tablespoons potato starch, or cornstarch

2 tablespoons fresh chopped sweet basil (or 2 teaspoons dried)
1 teaspoon fresh chopped thyme (or ½ teaspoon dried thyme)
1 teaspoon fresh chopped oregano (or ½ teaspoon dried oregano)
½ cup chopped green bell pepper
2 tablespoons chopped parsley (or 1 tablespoon dried parsley)
1 2-ounce jar pimiento, chopped (or ½ cup green chiles)
½ cup chopped green onions

8 egg whites

Blend the first 6 ingredients in a blender or food processor until smooth. Pour mixture into a large mixing bowl, then stir in herbs and vegetables. Beat egg whites in an electric mixer until stiff but not dry. Lightly fold beaten egg whites into cheese-herb mixture in bowl. Spread into a 2-quart souffle dish and bake at 350° for 35 to 45 minutes or until brown and raised. Serve immediately. Serves 4.

Crockpot Carrot-Sweet Potato Tzimmes (GF)

2 large bunches of carrots, sliced
4 medium sweet potatoes, peeled and cut into pieces
1 small onion, chopped
1 ½ cups water
1 pound prunes (only if you can find unsulfered prunes) (optional)

4 egg whites
½ cup honey
⅛ teaspoon ground pepper
1 teaspoon coriander

Mix together first 5 ingredients in a large crockpot. Set temperature on high, and cook for 8 to 10 hours. Tzimmes can also be baked covered in a 350° oven for 3 hours. After 1 ½ hours check to see if additional water is needed, and add an additional ½ cup of water if dry. One-half hour before serving whisk the last 4 ingredients, and stir this mixture into the tzimmes. Cook (or bake uncovered) for one-half hour longer. Serves 6 to 8.

Potato-Cheese Casserole

Potatoes and cheese are made for each other. Au grain potatoes are usually very rich, with butter, cheese and rich milk or cream. This recipe tastes rich and delicious with very little cholesterol, fat and salt. Serve this entree with a large raw vegetable salad.

6 medium potatoes, white rose or other cooking potatoes, scrubbed, whole unpeeled

2 cups low-fat cottage cheese
2 tablespoons whole wheat flour
2 tablespoons onion powder
¼ teaspoon garlic powder
¼ teaspoon black pepper
½ cup non-fat milk

sprinkle of paprika

Continues on the next page

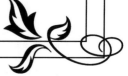

Boil potatoes until tender. Cool slightly in cold water. Meanwhile puree next 6 ingredients in a blender or food processor until smooth. Peel potatoes and slice them into ¼-inch slices. Arrange slices in a 9x9-inch non-stick baking pan and pour cottage cheese mixture over potato slices. Sprinkle with paprika. Bake in 350° oven for 20 minutes, then place casserole under the broiler for 5 to 10 minutes until golden brown and bubbly. Serves 3 to 4.

Chili-Bell Pepper Quiche

Imagine—a beautiful spicy quiche that is low in cholesterol and salt. This is it! With a salad and cooked vegetable you have a lovely healthy meal.

1 small onion, diced
2 cloves garlic, minced

1 cup chopped red and green bell peppers
2 heaping tablespoons green chili peppers, chopped (or ½ fresh jalapeno pepper, chopped)

2 ½ cups low-fat cottage cheese

6 egg whites
1 ½ teaspoons onion powder
⅛ teaspoon pepper
dash of nutmeg
1 tablespoon whole wheat pastry flour

sprinkle of paprika for top

Saute onions and garlic in a non-stick frying pan until brown and softened. Add 1 or 2 tablespoons of water as needed to keep onions from sticking and burning. Stir in bell peppers and chili peppers and fry until moisture is gone. Meanwhile whip cottage cheese in blender or food processor. Add egg whites, onion powder, pepper, nutmeg and flour and blend for ½ minute longer. Pour cottage cheese mixture into a large mixing bowl. Stir in sauteed vegetables, and pour mixture into prepared Grape-Nuts Crust. Sprinkle top with paprika. Bake in 350° oven for approximately 25 to 35 minutes or until set. Allow quiche to cool for 10 minutes before serving. Serve warm. Serves 4.

Grape-Nuts Onion-Chili Crust

½ cup Grape-Nuts cereal
1 ½ tablespoons water
1 teaspoon onion powder
½ teaspoon chili powder

Place 4 crust ingredients in a 9-inch glass oven-proof pie plate. Mix together to moisten cereal, then pat cereal evenly on bottom. Bake in a 350° oven for 7 minutes.

Note: –   This quiche can be made earlier in the day and refrigerated until 30 minutes before serving. Reheat quiche in a 300° oven for 20 to 30 minutes, just until heated through.

Leek and Cheese Quiche with Herbs

This quiche has a delicious flavor and you don't have to worry about the cheese, egg yolks, and cream in regular quiches.

3 cups sliced leeks, white part only (sliced very thin by hand)
½ cup thinly sliced celery
½ cup thinly sliced carrots
½ cup chopped onion
2 cloves garlic, minced
1 bay leaf
½ teaspoon dry mustard
½ teaspoon thyme
½ teaspoon basil
dash of nutmeg
dash of cayenne
¼ cup water

Continues on the next page

2 ½ cups low-fat cottage cheese
1 teaspoon onion powder
½ teaspoon garlic powder
6 egg whites
1 tablespoon whole wheat pastry flour

sprinkle of thyme and paprika for top

Saute first 12 ingredients in a non-stick frying pan until moisture is absorbed. Whip cottage cheese in a blender or food processor until smooth. Blend in egg whites, flour and seasonings for ½ minute longer, then pour mixture into a large mixing bowl and stir in sauteed vegetables. Pour mixture into prepared Grape-Nuts Crust, and sprinkle top with thyme and paprika. Bake in a 350° oven for 25 to 35 minutes. Allow quiche to cool for 10 minutes before serving. Serve warm. Serves 4.

Grape-Nuts Crust with Thyme

½ cup Grape-Nuts cereal
1 ½ tablespoons water
½ teaspoon garlic powder
½ teaspoon onion powder
½ teaspoon thyme

Place 5 crust ingredients in a 9-inch glass oven-proof pie plate. Mix together to moisten crust, then pat mixture on the bottom and bake in a 350° oven for 7 minutes.

Spicy Layered Lentil-Rice Casserole with Spicy Cumin-Mustard Sauce (GF)

Bean and grain combinations are an excellent source of protein. This colorful casserole makes a nutritious and delicious, non-dairy meal. Serve it with a large raw vegetable salad.

Continues on the next page

4 cups cooked lentils (2 cups raw lentils cooked until soft in 4 cups water with ½ medium onion)

2 teaspoons wine vinegar

1 tablespoon cumin

1 teaspoon dried, ground mustard

4 cups cooked Basic Brown Rice (see chapter on Basics)

½ cup chopped onion

¼ cup chopped green onion

½ medium-sized green bell pepper, chopped

½ medium-sized red bell pepper, chopped

½ teaspoon garlic powder

2 ½ cups Spicy Cumin-Mustard Sauce

Mix lentils, vinegar and spices together in a small bowl. In another bowl mix together next 6 ingredients and set aside. Layer the casserole in a 9x9-inch non-stick or glass oven-proof baking pan as follows: Spread ½ cup Spicy Cumin-Mustard Sauce on the bottom of the baking pan, then spread ½ of lentils over sauce, spread ½ of rice mixture over lentils, and spread ½ cup of sauce over rice layer. Repeat this process ending with ½ cup of sauce on top. Bake casserole in a 425° oven for 1 hour 15 minutes or until hot, crusty and bubbly. Before serving heat remaining cup of Spicy Cumin-Mustard Sauce and spoon it over each portion. Serves 6.

Spicy Cumin-Mustard Sauce (GF)

¾ cup tomato puree

1 ¾ cups water

1 ½ teaspoons chili powder

2 teaspoons onion powder

⅛ teaspoon pepper

1⁄16 teaspoon cayenne

½ teaspoon garlic powder

1 ½ teaspoons cumin

½ teaspoon dried mustard

Continues on the next page

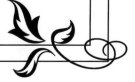

1 tablespoon potato or cornstarch
2 tablespoons cold water

Cook first 9 ingredients in a 2-quart saucepan over medium heat until sauce comes to a boil. Reduce heat and simmer for 10 minutes. In a cup dissolve starch in water and gradually, add to sauce, stirring constantly until sauce thickens a little. Yields 2 ½ cups of sauce.

Eggplant Cheese Casserole
with Caraway Seeds

If you like eggplant and caraway seeds you'll enjoy this tasty, easy-to-prepare and nutritious casserole.

4 cups pared, cubed eggplant
½ medium onion, finely chopped
½ cup water

4 egg whites, slightly beaten
4 slices rye bread with caraway seeds, broken into small pieces (or 1 ½ cups whole grain
    bread crumbs)
½ cup non-fat milk
1 teaspoon onion powder
⅛ teaspoon ground pepper
1 cup low-fat cottage cheese, whipped

sprinkle of paprika on top

Steam eggplant and onion in water, covered, until eggplant is tender, for about 7 minutes. Remove to a large mixing bowl. Stir in next 6 ingredients. Spread evenly in a 9x9-inch non-stick or glass oven-proof baking pan. Sprinkle with paprika and bake uncovered in a 350° oven for 25 minutes. Serves 3 or 4.

Note: – *If rye bread with caraway seeds is not available, use any whole grain bread and add 1 teaspoon of caraway seeds. Try to use bread made without salt, fat or sugar whenever possible. Pritikin rye and wheat breads are available in many parts of the country, made without any sugar, salt or fat.*

Kasha with Mushrooms, Walnuts, and Onions (Buckwheat Groats)

This dish is truly a hearty, wholesome protein meal and an excellent entree. Buckwheat is the highest protein of all grains, especially when combined with nuts and served with a dollop of Creamy Cottage Cheese Topping.

2 large onions, finely chopped
4 stalks celery, chopped

1 cup kasha (buckwheat groats)
2 egg whites

2 cups boiling water

½ pound mushrooms, sliced
½ cup chopped walnuts
¼ teaspoon ground pepper
1 teaspoon dill weed
1 teaspoon cider vinegar

1 cup Creamy Cottage Cheese Topping or Mock Sour Cream, optional, (see chapter on Basics)

Saute onions and celery in a large non-stick frying pan until onions are brown. Remove to a plate or bowl. Mix together kasha and egg whites in a small bowl until kasha is well coated. Heat frying pan again and fry kasha kernels, stirring constantly until kernels are separated and dry. Stir in onion-celery mixture and boiling water. Reduce heat, cover, and simmer for approximately 15 minutes, until liquid is absorbed. Then stir in next 5 ingredients and cook one minute longer. Serves 3 to 4.

Thanksgiving Vegi Turkey Loaf
with Thick Mushroom Gravy- Gluten Free Option

No one will miss a turkey when they can enjoy this marvelous, nutritious loaf with thick luscious Mushroom Gravy. To make your holiday meal even more festive, serve this entree with Yummy Yam Meringue Casserole, Orange Cranberry Relish and a steamed green vegetable.

Vegi Turkey Loaf:
½ bunch celery, diced
6 large carrots, shredded
2 ½ onions, chopped
6 cloves garlic, minced
3 tomatoes, chopped
1 cup water
2 teaspoons oregano
1 teaspoon sage
1 teaspoon rosemary
1 teaspoon black pepper
¼ teaspoon cayenne
2 ½ cups brown rice, raw
5 cups water
1 tablespoon onion powder
2 teaspoons celery seed
½ teaspoon black pepper
½ cup white wine or 2 tablespoons wine vinegar

4 cups toasted whole wheat or Gluten Free bread crumbs
⅓ cup walnuts, chopped
⅓ cup almonds, chopped
4 cups low-fat cottage cheese
1 tablespoon onion powder
1 tablespoon garlic powder

Continues on the next page

To prepare loaf: Cook first 11 ingredients in a large saucepan covered over medium-low heat for approximately 30 minutes or until celery is soft. Reserve 1 ½ cups of the liquid from vegetables for topping and use the remaining juice and vegetables in the loaf.

Cook rice in water, wine and seasonings, covered, until water is absorbed, for approximately 45 minutes.

Mix together all ingredients for loaf in a large bowl or pot. Check seasonings. You may wish to add more onion powder or pepper. A little dill may be added. Form into one loaf. Place loaf in a 10x15-inch non-stick jelly roll pan or large roasting pan.

Nut Topping for Vegi Turkey Loaf:
1 ½ cups ground pecans
1 ½ cups ground almonds
4 cups toasted whole wheat bread crumbs
1 cup low-fat cottage cheese, whipped
1 ½ cups liquid reserved from cooked vegetables

Mix together all the topping ingredients with enough liquid from the cooked vegetables to make it like a dough. Pat mixture all over loaf to cover well with fingers, a little at a time.

Bake loaf in a 375° oven, covered, for 30 minutes, then uncovered for 30 to 45 minutes or until nut topping is golden brown. Serve with Mushroom Gravy. Serves 12 to 16.

Note: – *The loaf, topping and gravy can be made earlier in the day and allowed to stand out of refrigerator for at least 2 hours before baking. I cook the rice, prepare the bread crumbs, and chop nuts the day before to save time.*

Thick Mushroom Gravy-(GF)

2 ½ onions, chopped
7 cloves garlic, minced
⅛ teaspoon black pepper
⅛ teaspoon oregano
pinch of thyme
pinch of cayenne

2 pounds mushrooms, sliced or crushed

Continues on the next page

1 cup low-fat cottage cheese
1 cup evaporated skimmed milk
¼ cup water

Saute first 6 ingredients in a large non-stick frying pan until onions are softened and lightly browned. Add 1 or 2 tablespoons of water as needed to keep mixture from sticking or burning. Stir in mushrooms and cook for 25 to 30 minutes over low heat, stirring occasionally. Cool slightly and puree half of the mushroom mixture. Stir in pureed mixture to the remaining portion in frying pan.

This much of the sauce can be prepared ahead of time and refrigerated. Before serving slowly heat mushroom-onion mixture in a large non-stick saucepan with cottage cheese, milk and water. Do not boil. Serve over each portion of Vegi Turkey. Yields 1-quart of sauce.

Oven-Baked Lima Bean-Potato Stew- (GF) (Cholent)

This satisfying, inexpensive and nutritious meal was prepared and baked by eastern European Jews in brick ovens on Friday afternoon and eaten on Saturday afternoon. Ours is made without fat, cholesterol or salt.

3 cups (or 1 pound) dried lima beans
water to cover

3 large onions, sliced
6 cloves garlic
6 stalks celery

4 large potatoes, peeled and cut in quarters
6 carrots cut in half
2 bay leaves
2 tablespoons dried parsley flakes
½ teaspoon pepper
2 teaspoons celery seed
1 tablespoon dried dill weed
3 tablespoons cider vinegar or wine vinegar

8 cups boiling water

Continues on the next page

Place beans and water in a large soup pot or Dutch oven. Bring beans to a boil, and cook them, covered, for 10 minutes. Remove pot from heat and allow beans to remain in hot water until cool or overnight. Discard bean liquid, rinse beans, and place them into a large bowl.

Brown onions, garlic and celery in same soup pot. Return beans to pot, stir in next 8 ingredients, then add boiling water. Cover tightly and bring to a boil

To finish cooking: Place bean stew in a 400° oven for ½ hour. Then turn oven to 250° and cook overnight and until noon of the next day. Cholent may also be cooked on the stove over a very low flame for 3 hours. Great care must be taken to see that beans do not burn. This stew can also be cooked in a large crockpot for 8 to 10 hours or until ready to serve. Serves 8.

Yummy Yam-Meringue Casserole

This recipe makes a great holiday buffet side dish or a delicious, unusual dessert. The yam layer can be made ahead of time.

Yam Layer
4 cups pureed yams or sweet potatoes
2 cups evaporated skimmed milk
2 tablespoons honey
2 teaspoons grated orange rind
½ teaspoon cardamom
½ teaspoon allspice
¼ teaspoon nutmeg
2 tablespoons whole wheat pastry flour
2 egg whites

Whisk all ingredients for yam layer until well mixed. Pour this mixture into a 2-quart souffle dish or an oven-proof bowl. Before serving bake yam layer in a 375° oven for 30 minutes. Meanwhile prepare the meringue.

Continues on the next page

Meringue:

4 egg whites

3 tablespoons honey

¼ teaspoon cardamom
¼ teaspoon coriander
⅛ teaspoon nutmeg

Beat egg whites in an electric mixer until foamy. Gradually beat in honey and continue beating until whites are stiff and shiny. Add spices. Remove souffle dish from oven. Pour meringue on top. Return casserole to oven and bake for 15 minutes longer or until meringue is lightly browned. Serves 8 to 10 small servings.

Steamy Baked Potatoes with Steamed Broccoli and Topped with Creamy Mushroom-Cheese-Wine Sauce (GF)

What could be more satisfying than a steaming hot potato, cut in half, piled high with lightly steamed broccoli and topped with a lovely mushroom-cheese sauce? The combination of these ingredients are very well balanced and nutritious.

2 large-sized baking potatoes, well scrubbed

1 10-ounce package of frozen broccoli spears

Creamy Mushroom Cheese Wine Sauce

Bake potatoes until soft. Steam broccoli until barely tender. Cut potatoes open, place broccoli in center and top with sauce. Serves 2.

Creamy Mushroom-Cheese-Wine Sauce (GF)

You can also use this sauce for egg white omelettes, crepes, or on top of cooked green beans or asparagus.

½ pound mushrooms, sliced
2 green onions, minced
2 tablespoons white wine
⅛ teaspoon black pepper

1 cup low-fat cottage cheese
1 teaspoon onion powder

Combine mushrooms, green onions, wine and pepper in non-stick frying pan. Cook just until moisture is gone, for approximately 5 to 8 minutes. Remove mushroom mixture to a plate or bowl. Heat the cottage cheese and onion powder in the same frying pan over medium heat just until cottage cheese melts. This takes only a few minutes. Do not boil. Stir in mushroom mixture and heat for a minute or two longer, just until heated through. Serves 2 or 3.

Stuffed Cabbage Boats with Sweet and Sour Sauce (GF)

This vegetable, rice and cheese entree has everything in it for a tasty, nutritious and satisfying meal.

1 medium head cabbage, cut in quarters
1 cup boiling water

3 cups cooked brown rice
1 small red bell pepper, or 1 2-ounce jar pimiento
1 teaspoon thyme
2 cups low-fat cottage cheese
1 teaspoon onion powder
⅛ teaspoon black pepper
½ cup Sweet and Sour Sauce

Continues on the next page

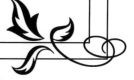

½ medium onion

2 cloves garlic

1 medium green bell pepper

½ cup Sweet and Sour Sauce for pan

½ cup Sweet and Sour Sauce for topping

In a large pot steam cabbage quarters, covered, in boiling water for 5 to 8 minutes or until a fork can pierce the cabbage. Remove a few of the inner leaves and reserve them for the rice stuffing. Mix together the next 7 ingredients in a large mixing bowl. Then chop onion, garlic, bell pepper and reserved cabbage leaves in a blender or food processor. Stir cabbage mixture into ingredients already in mixing bowl.

To assemble: Separate each cabbage quarter into two boats. Spread ½ cup of Sweet and Sour Sauce on the bottom of a 9x13-inch non-stick or glass oven-proof baking pan. Stuff cabbage boats and arrange them over sauce in baking pan. Pour additional sauce on top and bake in a 350° oven for 30 minutes or until hot and light brown. Serves 6 to 8.

Sweet and Sour Sauce:
1 ½ cups tomato puree
¼ cup cider vinegar
2 tablespoons concentrated apple juice
¼ teaspoon black pepper
¼ cup black raisins

Simmer ingredients together in a non-stick saucepan for 15 minutes.

Scrumptuous Spinach Soy Burgers (GF)

These luscious burgers can be eaten on a bun or in a pita with a slice of onion, tomato, lettuce (or sprouts), salt-free mustard, and Homemade Chili Sauce or Mickey's Tangy Relish. They can also be eaten without a bun as a protein entree, or taken for lunches straight from the freezer. In storing them in refrigerator or freezer separate patties so they won't stick together.

Continues on the next page

4 cups cooked and drained soybeans

1 10-ounce package chopped spinach, thawed, not drained or squeezed out

2 egg whites

2 cups wheat flakes or cornflakes (GF)

3 green onions

½ medium green bell pepper

2 teaspoons thyme

1 teaspoon garlic powder

¼ teaspoon ground pepper

4 teaspoons onion powder

2 cups low-fat cottage cheese

Chop all ingredients in a food processor or blender, in batches if necessary, only until beans are mashed. Pour mixture into a bowl. Heat a large non-stick frying pan or griddle, and drop by large spoonfuls, shaping patties as large as desired. Fry over medium heat until brown on both sides. Patties can also be baked on one side only in a 400° oven in a non-stick 10x15-inch jelly roll pan for approximately 15 minutes or until patties are firm. Loosen patties gently. Yields 8 patties.

Easy Spinach-Cheese Casserole

This is a favorite of our family, and so easy to prepare.

2 cups low-fat cottage cheese

1 package frozen chopped spinach, thawed, and drained but not squeezed out

6 egg whites

2 tablespoons whole wheat pastry flour

1 ½ teaspoons onion powder

⅛ teaspoon black pepper

Mix together all ingredients in a mixing bowl. Bake in a 1 ½ quart casserole dish for 30 minutes, or just until set in a 350° oven. Serves 2.

Note: – *Recipe can be doubled or tripled as a party dish and baked in a 9x13-inch non-stick or glass oven-proof baking dish, for approximately 45 minutes to 1 hour.*

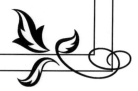

Spicy Stuffed Acorn Squash (GF)

The exotic spices in this recipe complement the naturally delicate flavor of the squash. This entree is easy to prepare and a real treat to eat.

2 small to medium acorn squash, cut in half, seeded
1 cup cooked brown rice
½ cup soft whole grain or Gluten Free bread crumbs
⅔ cup low-fat cottage cheese
¼ cup black raisins
1 medium tart apple, chopped
¼ cup onion, finely chopped
1⁄16 teaspoon cayenne
2 teaspoons curry powder
1 teaspoon coriander
3 tablespoons concentrated apple juice

4 teaspoons concentrated apple juice reserved for top
sprinkle of coriander for top

Place halves of acorn squash, cavity facing down, in a 9x13-inch baking pan with ½ inch of water. Bake in a 350° oven for 30 minutes or until squash is tender when center is pierced with a fork. While squash is baking mix together the next 10 ingredients. Stuff the squash halves. Pour 1 teaspoon apple juice over each, sprinkle with coriander, and bake in a 350° oven for approximately 25 to 30 minutes or until hot and light brown on top. Serves 4.

Easy Potato Pancakes (or Potato Pudding)

6 medium white rose potatoes, or other cooking potatoes, unpeeled, cut into 12 pieces
1 small white onion, cut into eighths
9 egg whites, unbeaten

Continues on the next page

2 tablespoons whole wheat flour

1 tablespoon onion powder

¼ teaspoon ground pepper

Grate the potatoes and onion with egg whites in batches in a blender or food processor, adding flour and seasonings to the last batch. Do not puree potatoes. Pour grated potato mixture into a large mixing bowl.

Spoon batter into a hot non-stick griddle or large frying pan, and fry until pancakes are brown on both sides. Serves 4.

Ratatouille (GF)

This succulent vegetable dish is excellent served over Basic Brown Rice or whole wheat pasta, or as a filling for crepes.

2 medium onions, sliced

3 cloves garlic, minced

1 teaspoon oregano

2 teaspoons thyme

1 medium eggplant, unpeeled, cubed

3 medium zucchini, sliced

8 medium tomatoes, diced

3 carrots, thinly sliced

3 celery stalks, sliced

2 tablespoons cider or wine vinegar

¼ cup pine nuts, or sunflower seeds

Fry sliced onions and chopped garlic, uncovered, until lightly browned in large non-stick frying pan that has a tight fitting lid. Add herbs to hot pan and stir for 30 seconds to release flavor from herbs. Stir in vegetables and vinegar, then cover tightly, and simmer vegetables over medium-low heat for 15 to 20 minutes.

Remove from flame. Sprinkle nuts or seeds on top of each serving. Serves 4 to 6.

Cheese-Corn-Pimiento-Rice Casserole

This delicious casserole is easy to prepare and it makes a very nutritious meal. Serve it with steamed carrots and a salad.

4 cups low-fat cottage cheese, whipped
6 egg whites
1 10-ounce frozen corn kernels, thawed and drained
2 teaspoons onion powder
¼ cup chopped fresh pimiento, or 1 2-ounce jar pimiento
¼ cup chopped green onions
2 tablespoons whole wheat pastry flour
2 cups cooked brown rice

Mix all ingredients together in a large mixing bowl. Spread evenly in a 9x9-inch non-stick or glass oven-proof baking dish and bake in a 350° oven for 30 to 40 minutes or until set and light brown on top. Do not overbake. Allow to set for 10 minutes and spoon to serve. Serves 4.

Succulent Vegetarian Low-Cal Moussaka (GF)

This succulent and exotic entree makes an excellent party or buffet dish. It is very low in cholesterol and salt and the aroma is divine as it bakes.

Moussaka:
1 ½ large onions, chopped
½ cup tomato puree

2 large firm eggplants, sliced thin
1 teaspoon onion powder
⅓ cup dry white wine

Continues on the next page

¾ teaspoon cinnamon
½ cup parsley, minced
⅛ teaspoon black pepper

2 tablespoons potato starch or cornstarch
2 tablespoons water or wine

Simmer onion with tomato puree in a large non-stick pot, covered, for 5 minutes. Stir in sliced eggplant, onion powder and wine to the tomato onion mixture, and simmer covered for 5 to 10 minutes longer, or until eggplant is barely tender but not overcooked. Add cinnamon, parsley and pepper to sauce. Mix together starch and water or wine, and gradually stir this mixture into sauteed eggplant until thickened. Spread eggplant mixture into a 9x13-inch glass oven-proof or non-stick baking pan. Set aside.

Cheese Topping:
1 ½ cups evaporated skimmed milk
½ cup water
¼ teaspoon white pepper
3 tablespoons whole wheat pastry flour or Gluten Free flour

2 cups low-fat cottage cheese
2 teaspoons onion powder
½ teaspoon nutmeg
4 egg whites

Whisk evaporated skimmed milk, water, white pepper and flour into mixing bowl. Pour this mixture into a non-stick sauce pan. Stir constantly over medium heat until mixture thickens. Remove from heat and let it cool slightly. Meanwhile whip cottage cheese with nutmeg and onion powder in a blender or food processor. Add egg whites and blend for a minute longer. Pour cottage cheese mixture into a large mixing bowl and stir in milk-flour mixture.

Spread cheese topping over casserole and bake in a 350° oven for approximately 45 minutes, or until top is golden brown. Remove from oven and let it cool for 15 minutes before serving. Serves 6 to 8.

Pimiento-Chile Quiche (GF)

This attractive quiche has an exciting flavor, and a lovely salmon color.

1 cup chopped onions
2 cloves garlic, minced
¼ cup water

2 ½ cups low-fat cottage cheese, whipped

1 4-ounce jar sliced pimientos
2 ounces canned diced green chiles
1 teaspoon onion powder
dash of nutmeg
½ teaspoon oregano
6 egg whites

1 heaping teaspoon oregano, crumbled

Saute onions and garlic in water in a non-stick frying pan until onions are soft and beginning to brown. Remove from heat and set aside.

Whip cottage cheese in a blender or food processor. Blend in next 6 ingredients for ½ minute longer, and pour into prepared Grape-Nuts Crust. Sprinkle with crumbled oregano.

Bake in a 350° oven for 30 to 35 minutes. Allow to cool for 10 minutes before slicing. Serves 4.

Grape-Nuts Crust with Oregano

¾ cup Grape-Nuts cereal
3 tablespoons water
1 teaspoon onion powder
½ teaspoon oregano

Continues on the next page

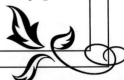

Combine 4 crust ingredients, and moisten cereal well. Pour into a 9-inch glass oven-proof pie plate, and pat mixture evenly on bottom. Partially bake crust for 7 minutes in a 350° oven.

Note: — *This quiche can be made earlier in the day and refrigerated until 30 minutes before serving. Reheat quiche in a 300° oven for 20 to 30 minutes, just until heated through.*

Crustless Zucchini Quiche with Dill

This low-calorie quiche is nutritious and delicious. You can eat as much as you like.

1 small onion, diced
2 cloves garlic, minced
4 green onions, stems and roots, chopped
¼ cup chopped red or green bell pepper

4 cups zucchini, sliced very thin

3 cups low-fat cottage cheese, whipped

½ teaspoon garlic powder
1 ½ teaspoons onion powder
⅛ teaspoon red pepper
2 teaspoons dill weed
dash of nutmeg
6 egg whites
1 tablespoon whole wheat pastry flour

Saute first 4 ingredients in a non-stick frying pan until brown and softened. Add 1 or 2 tablespoons water as needed to keep onions from sticking and burning. Stir in zucchini slices until zucchini is slightly softened, then remove from heat.

Whip cottage cheese in blender or food processor until smooth. In a large mixing bowl whisk the remaining 7 ingredients. Stir in the cheese mixture and zucchini-onion mixture, and pour into a 9x9-inch non-stick or glass oven-proof baking dish. Bake quiche in a 325° oven for 30 to 35 minutes or until set. Allow quiche to cool for 10 minutes before serving. Serves 4 to 6.

Gourmet Mushroom-Cheese Casserole (GF)

This delightful tasting gourmet casserole should be prepared the day before and baked before serving. It is sure to bring raves. You might wish to double the recipe and take it to a pot-luck supper.

1 onion, minced
2 cloves garlic, minced
1 pound mushrooms, sliced
1 ½ teaspoons vegetarian-herbal seasoning (without salt)
dash cayenne
dash nutmeg
dash white or black pepper

6 egg whites
2 cups low-fat cottage cheese
1 cup evaporated skimmed milk
4 slices soft wheat bread (or 2 soft whole wheat rolls or Gluten free bread), cut into small
    cubes

Saute onion, garlic, mushrooms and seasoning until brown in a non-stick frying pan. Stir in a little water as needed to keep mushrooms from sticking. Mix together remaining ingredients in a mixing bowl, stir in mushroom mixture, and spread into a 1 ½-quart souffle dish. Allow to stand for at least 5 hours before baking (or better still prepare the day before).

   Bake in 350° oven for 30 minutes or just until set. Do not overbake. Serves 2 or 3.

Note: –   *If recipe is doubled or tripled, bake casserole for approximately 1 hour, or just until set. Do not overbake.*

Lentil Roast with Mushroom Sauce

This mouth-watering entree with this delectable sauce makes a marvelous, healthful, well balanced entree.

Continues on the next page

2 cups cooked lentils (1 cup raw lentils cooked in 2 cups water with 2 teaspoons onion
  powder)

½ cup chopped nuts

6 egg whites

1 cup evaporated skimmed milk (or double strength reconstituted non-fat milk powder)

1 ½ cups whole wheat bread crumbs or crushed corn flakes, or wheat flakes

1 teaspoon dill weed

½ teaspoon sage

1 tablespoon apple cider or wine vinegar

1 small onion finely chopped

1 cup grated carrots

1 cup grated celery

1 teaspoon oregano, crumbled for top

Mix together all ingredients except oregano. Pour mixture into a 9x9-inch non-stick or glass oven-proof baking pan. Sprinkle oregano on top and bake in a 350° oven for 35 to 45 minutes or until golden brown. Serve hot with Mushroom Sauce, or chill and cut into slices for sandwich filling. Serves 4.

Mushroom Sauce (GF)

1 small onion, chopped

2 cloves garlic, minced

2 tablespoons water

½ pound mushrooms, chopped

½ cup low-fat cottage cheese

¼ cup evaporated skimmed milk

pinch of black pepper

pinch of oregano

pinch of thyme

pinch of cayenne

Continues on the next page

In a non-stick frying pan saute onion and garlic in water until soft and lightly brown. Add mushrooms and cook over low heat for 15 to 20 minutes, stirring occasionally. Before serving add remaining ingredients. Heat slowly until cheese melts. Do not allow sauce to boil. Serve at once. Yields 1 cup of sauce.

Luscious Lentil Burgers (GF)

What a pleasure it is to enjoy healthy vegi-burgers with all the trimmings. These great tasting burgers have as much protein as meat burgers, and with very little cholesterol or fat.

2 cups raw lentils (rinsed)
4 cups water
1 medium onion, chopped
2 bay leaves
1 teaspoon celery seed

2 cups low-fat cottage cheese
½ teaspoon black pepper
1 ½ cups wheat flakes or cornflakes (GF)
1 teaspoon oregano
1 teaspoon curry powder
2 teaspoons cumin powder
½ teaspoon garlic powder
¼ cup raw sunflower seeds, or sesame seeds

Cook first 5 ingredients in a large pot for approximately 30 minutes or until water is absorbed. Remove from heat and stir in remaining ingredients. Drop by large spoonfuls in a non-stick 10x15-inch jelly roll pan. Flatten and shape into patties, and bake on one side for 15 minutes or until burgers are firm. Burgers can also be fried in a non-stick frying pan or griddle until brown on both sides. Yields 8 patties.

Flo's Farmers Chop Suey (GF)

This crunchy salad makes a delicious buffet dish, or a satisfying light lunch or dinner. It is especially refreshing in warm weather.

3 carrots, sliced
3 stalks celery, sliced
1 cucumber, cut in half and sliced
4 sprigs of parsley, chopped
3 green onions, chopped
5 or 6 radishes, sliced

2 cups low-fat cottage cheese, whipped
½ cup plain non-fat yogurt
1 teaspoon onion powder

2 tomatoes, cut in wedges

Mix together chopped vegetables, reserving tomato wedges for decoration. Combine cottage cheese, yogurt and onion powder and fold into vegetables. Garnish with tomatoes and refrigerate until serving. Serves 3 or 4.

Oriental Tofu-Vegetable Delight with Fat-Free Fried Brown Rice (GF)

The flavor of fresh ginger in this recipe adds a delightful touch to this healthy and substantial meal. Serve over Fat-Free Fried Brown Rice, and top with Mock Soy Sauce.

2 pieces of fresh ginger root (each piece ½-inch thick and 1-inch round), peeled
2 cloves of garlic
½ medium onion

½ cup Mock Soy Sauce or Gluten free soy sauce (see chapter on Basics)

Continues on the next page

1 pound firm tofu, rinsed and patted dry

½ medium onion, chopped
½ medium cabbage, cut into long strips ½-inch wide
4 green onions, cut into pieces 2-inches long
½ large red bell pepper, cut into strips
½ large green bell pepper, cut into strips

Grate ginger root, garlic and onion in a blender or food processor. Place this mixture into a medium-sized mixing bowl. Stir in ½ cup of Mock Soy Sauce and mix well. Cut tofu into 1-inch cubes. Toss the tofu cubes in the Mock Soy Sauce mixture and marinate for several hours. Turn at least once.

Prepare vegetables and set aside. Twenty minutes before serving, saute marinated tofu along with marinade in a large non-stick frying pan over medium heat until most of the moisture is absorbed. Remove tofu from pan and set aside.

Right before serving stir-fry vegetables in the same pan for a few minutes until vegetables are hot, but not wilted. Stir in tofu. Heat and serve over rice. Serves 2 to 3.

Fat-Free Fried Brown Rice (GF)

2 to 3 cups of Basic Cooked Brown Rice (see chapter on Basics)
4 green onions, chopped
½ medium onion, chopped
¼ cup Mock Soy Sauce (see chapter on Basics)

Heat all ingredients in a non-stick frying pan, stirring occasionally for 10 to 12 minutes, or until rice is hot. Serves 2 to 3.

Tofu "Pepper Steak" with Easy Potato Pancakes (GF)

If you want a real treat, try this tofu "pepper steak." It goes great with Easy Potato Pancakes topped with Homemade Apple Butter.

Continues on the next page

1 medium onion, minced

4 cloves of garlic, minced

½ cup Mock Soy Sauce (see chapter on Basics)

2 pounds firm tofu, drained and patted dry

2 green bell peppers, cut into strips

2 medium onions, sliced thin

1 cup tomato puree

¼ cup water

2 bay leaves

2 sprigs of green celery leaves

½ teaspoon thyme

2 tablespoons chopped fresh parsley

Mix together first 3 ingredients. Cut each pound of tofu into steaks each approximately ½-inch thick. Pour half of the Mock Soy Sauce mixture in the bottom of a 9x13-inch glass oven-proof baking dish. Arrange tofu steaks over marinade and pour the remainder on top of each slice. Allow tofu steaks to marinate for several hours, or longer.

One-half hour before serving saute tofu steaks in marinade until brown on both sides. Remove tofu from pan and set aside. Simmer all remaining ingredients in the same frying pan for 5 minutes. Return tofu steaks to the pan and simmer slowly for 15 minutes. Serve tofu steaks with the vegetables and sauce. Serves 4.

Scrambled Tofu Jalapeno (GF)

This is surprisingly good and fun to eat. For folks who don't or can't eat eggs, it's a special treat. Turmeric gives the tofu the color of scrambled eggs. All the vegetables except for tomatoes can be chopped in the food processor.

1 pound firm tofu, rinsed well and dried

½ small green bell pepper, chopped

½ small red bell pepper, chopped

½ jalapeno pepper, chopped

2 small tomatoes, chopped coarsely

Continues on the next page

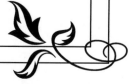

2 tablespoons chopped parsley

2 green onions, chopped

1 teaspoon onion powder

⅛ teaspoon black pepper

¼ teaspoon turmeric

Mash tofu with a fork into the consistency of scrambled eggs. Stir in the remaining ingredients. Slowly simmer all ingredients in a non-stick frying pan, covered, for 10 minutes. Then simmer uncovered for 10 minutes. Serves 3 or 4 people.

Vegi Bean and Cheese Enchiladas (GF)

At last! If you like Mexican food, try these low-fat, low-cholesterol, low-salt, lard-free Mexican enchiladas. They're delicious and wholesome.

2 cups Home-Made Enchilada Sauce (see chapter on Basics)

6 corn tortillas (made without preservatives or lard)
1 ½ cups Spicy Refried Beans (see chapter on Basics)

1 ½ cups low-fat cottage cheese

½ medium onion, chopped

¼ medium onion, chopped and reserved for topping

Pour 1 cup of enchilada sauce on the bottom of a 9x13-inch non-stick baking pan. Fill center of each tortilla with a generous heaping tablespoon of beans, a generous heaping tablespoon of cottage cheese, and a tablespoon of chopped onions. Roll up tortillas and place seam side down on top of sauce. Pour remaining sauce over enchiladas, and sprinkle chopped onion over the top.

Bake enchiladas in a 450° oven for approximately 30 to 35 minutes, or until top is crisp, sauce bubbly, and cheese begins to melt. Serves 3 to 4.

Tofu "Liver" Steak with Oven-Baked French Fries (GF)

Wow! What a dinner, and all without a trace of cholesterol. We suggest you serve it with Homemade Chili Sauce on the side.

1 medium onion, minced
4 cloves of garlic, minced
double recipe of Mock Soy Sauce (see chapter on Basics)

2 pounds firm tofu, drained and patted dry

3 large onions, sliced thin
¼ teaspoon pepper

Mix together first 3 ingredients. Cut each pound of tofu into steaks approximately ½-inch thick. Pour half the Mock Soy Sauce mixture in the bottom of a 9x13-inch glass baking dish. Arrange the tofu slices over marinade and pour the remainder over top. Allow slices to marinate for several hours or longer.

One-half hour before dinner saute tofu steaks and marinade in a large non-stick frying pan over medium heat, until tofu is brown on both sides. Remove from pan and set aside. Saute sliced onions and pepper in the same pan over medium-high heat until brown, stirring frequently. Return tofu to pan and simmer for 5 minutes. Serve tofu "liver" steaks with sliced onions on top. Serves 4.

Oven-Baked French Fries (GF)

4 medium potatoes, scrubbed, unpeeled

2 teaspoons onion powder

Cut potatoes lengthwise into fries. Sprinkle onion powder over fries and toss until mixed. Spread fries in a non-stick jelly roll pan and bake in a 450° oven, for approximately 15 minutes. Turn potatoes after they are brown on one side, and bake for an additional 10 to 15 minutes or until potatoes are tender and brown. Serves 2 to 4.

Stuffed Bell Peppers with Mushrooms and Curry (GF)

This entree makes a very healthy, tasty and attractive meal. We prepare this when peppers are in season.

1 cup uncooked brown rice
2 cups water
½ teaspoon celery seed
2 teaspoons onion powder

4 large bell peppers, halved lengthwise

½ pound mushrooms
2 large green onions or 3 small ones
6 sprigs of parsley
1 medium onion

2 cups low-fat cottage cheese
¼ teaspoon black pepper
2 teaspoons curry powder

½ cup tomato puree for bottom of baking pan

½ cup tomato puree for topping
1 teaspoon crushed oregano for topping

Cook rice and seasonings for approximately 35 minutes or until water is absorbed. Meanwhile cut bell peppers and parboil them in vegetable steamer for 10 minutes. Set peppers aside to cool.

Chop the next 4 ingredients in a blender or food processor. Do not puree. In a large mixing bowl place cottage cheese, curry and pepper, and stir in rice and mushroom mixtures. Spread tomato puree on the bottom of a 9x13-inch non-stick baking pan. Stuff peppers and arrange them on top of sauce. Extra stuffing can be placed between peppers. Spoon tomato puree for topping over stuffed peppers and sprinkle crushed oregano on top. Bake in a 350° oven for approximately 30 to 45 minutes or until well heated through. Serves 6.

Colorful Curried Vegetables over Fancy Wild and Brown Rice (GF)

This colorful party dish is exotically spiced and very nutritious. It is sure to bring raves, yet it contains no cholesterol. It is the perfect dish to serve for a holiday buffet.

Colorful Curried Vegetables:
1 onion, coarsely chopped
2 cloves garlic, minced

2 large boiling potatoes, peeled, cut into bite-size pieces
2 large tomatoes, chopped
½ green bell pepper, chopped
2 zucchini, sliced
2 cups thinly sliced carrots
2 teaspoons curry powder
1 teaspoon cumin
½ cup black raisins

¼ cup wine vinegar
2 tablespoons concentrated apple juice

1 10-ounce package frozen peas, thawed
1 10-ounce package frozen baby lima beans, thawed

Brown onion and garlic in a large non-stick frying pan, stirring occasionally. When the pan gets dry, stir in the next 8 ingredients. Saute vegetables for 5 minutes uncovered. Add vinegar and apple juice, cover, and allow vegetables to simmer over medium heat, stirring occasionally for approximately 20 minutes, or until vegetables are tender. Add peas and beans during the last 3 minutes of cooking. Serve over Fancy Wild and Brown Rice. Serves 6.

Continues on the next page

Fancy Wild and Brown Rice:

½ cup raw wild rice, pre-soaked according to instruction on package

2 cups raw brown rice

5 cups water

¾ cup dry white wine

½ teaspoon coriander

¼ teaspoon ground pepper

1 large onion, chopped

½ cup slivered almonds

1 pound mushrooms, sliced

¼ cup chopped green onions

¼ cup concentrated apple juice

2 tablespoons honey

1 tablespoon curry powder

Bring first 6 ingredients to a boil in a soup pot. Cook for approximately 40 to 45 minutes, or until water is absorbed. Meanwhile saute onion without oil in a non-stick frying pan. When liquid rendered is absorbed, add sliced mushrooms, almonds and green onions. Saute until moisture is absorbed. Stir in this mixture to cooked rice, along with apple juice, honey and curry powder. Remove rice mixture from heat and set aside. Heat before serving over low heat. Serves 6.

Note: – *Rice can be prepared earlier in the day and heated before serving. Sprinkle with a few drops of water before reheating.*

Rice-Nut Loaf with Quick Curry Cheese Sauce (GF)

This healthy and satisfying loaf will delight your taste buds and warm your tummy. Serve with Curry Cheese Sauce to create a nutritious protein entree.

2 cups cooked brown rice

1 cup soft wholegrain or Gluten free bread crumbs

1 cup chopped nuts

½ medium onion, finely chopped

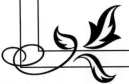

2 green onions, chopped
½ bell pepper, chopped
1 teaspoon thyme
⅛ teaspoon pepper
1 egg white
2 to 4 tablespoons non-fat milk

Mix together all ingredients, using just enough milk to hold mixture together. Shape into a loaf in a 9x13-inch non-stick baking pan and bake in a 375° oven for approximately 35 minutes, or until loaf is golden brown. Serves 3 or 4.

Quick Curry-Cheese Sauce (GF)

2 tablespoons evaporated skimmed milk
1 cup low-fat cottage cheese
1 teaspoon onion powder
2 teaspoons curry powder
dash of cayenne

Heat all ingredients together in a non-stick frying pan or saucepan stirring constantly until the cheese melts and the sauce begins to turn a little deeper color yellow. Do not allow sauce to boil. Serve at once. Yields 1 cup of sauce.

DESSERTS

Desserts

Finally, here are recipes for desserts that are divine, rich-tasting, beautiful to look at, AND "guilt-free."

Imagine, for example, a feather light dessert cake roll filled with creamy custard...made without cream, butter, egg yolks or sugar; and a golden brown, tall apple cake sweetened only with fruit and fruit juice; and luscious low-fat creamy cheesecakes, moist rich cakes, brownies, pies, dessert souffles, and wholegrain crunchy cookies to be enjoyed by you and your loved ones.

Pumpkin Spice Cake

This delightfully moist cake is both nutritious and delicious.

1 ½ cups honey
1 cup evaporated skimmed milk
8 egg whites
2 cups canned pumpkin puree
1 tablespoon cinnamon
1 teaspoon nutmeg
1 teaspoon ginger
¼ teaspoon cloves
⅔ cup water
1 tablespoon oil

3 ¾ cups whole wheat flour
1 tablespoon baking soda
1 teaspoon baking powder

Whisk first 10 ingredients in a large mixing bowl. Mix together flour, soda and baking powder and add, all at once, whisking just until blended. Do not overmix. Spread batter evenly in a 10-inch tube pan. Bake in a 350° oven for 1 hour or just until cake tests done. Do not overbake. Serves 10 to 12.

Viennese Apple Cake

This healthy dessert has all the appeal and delicious taste of old world baking without the negatives. If you love apples you'll flip over this one.

Apple Filling:
10 medium-sized Delicious apples, unpeeled and sliced thin in food processor or by hand
1 tablespoon cinnamon
½ cup concentrated apple juice

Continues on the next page

Cake Batter:
½ cup honey
2 egg whites
¾ cup evaporated skimmed milk
1 teaspoon cinnamon

1 ½ cups whole wheat flour
2 teaspoons baking powder

Topping:
1 cup Grape-Nuts cereal
1 cup chopped walnuts
2 teaspoons cinnamon
½ cup concentrated apple juice

2 egg whites
¼ cup evaporated skimmed milk

To prepare apple filling: Place apple slices, juice and cinnamon in a large bowl. Toss well and set aside.

To prepare cake batter: In another mixing bowl whisk the first 4 ingredients. Mix flour and baking powder together and add, all at once, whisking just until blended. Do not overbeat. Spread batter evenly in a 9x13-inch non-stick baking pan. Arrange the sliced apples on top of the cake batter.

To prepare topping: In a smaller bowl mix the first 4 topping ingredients together and sprinkle topping over apple slices. Then beat egg whites and milk together and pour mixture evenly over topping.

Bake in a 400° oven for 45 minutes or until cake is golden brown. Serve warm or cold. Serves 10 to 12.

Giant Apple Party Cake

The aroma of this cake baking is marvelous. You can feel very proud serving this beautiful, healthy and delicious cake.

Continues on the next page

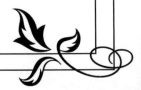

Cake Batter:

8 egg whites

½ cup evaporated skimmed milk

½ cup concentrated apple juice

1 teaspoon cinnamon

2 teaspoons vanilla

½ cup honey

1 teaspoon coriander

3 cups whole wheat pastry flour

1 tablespoon baking powder

2 teaspoons baking soda

Whisk first 7 ingredients in a large mixing bowl. Mix together flour, baking powder and soda and add, all at once, whisking just until blended. Set aside.

Apple Layers:

9 large Delicious apples, unpeeled, sliced thin in food processor or by hand (12 cups sliced apples)

½ cup concentrated apple juice

3 tablespoons cinnamon

1 teaspoon coriander

Toss together sliced apples, juice and spices. Set aside.

Cereal-Nut Layers:

2 cups Grape-Nuts cereal

1 cup chopped walnuts (optional)

½ cup walnut chunks for top

Mix together cereal and the chopped walnuts and set aside.

To assemble: In a 10-inch tube pan assemble cake as follows: one-third cereal-nut mixture on bottom of pan, one-third apple slices and one-third batter. Repeat these layers twice, ending with batter on top. Sprinkle top with the walnut chunks, pressing nuts gently down into batter.

Bake cake in a 350° oven for 1 hour and 50 minutes to 2 hours. If cake is browning too much on top, cover with foil last 15 minutes. After cake is cool it can be stored in refrigerator or freezer. Serves 10 to 12.

Fruit Sweetened Apple Ring Cake

So delicious and without any sweetners except apple juice. There's very low fat, cholesterol or salt. You won't miss all the calories and the taste is great.

8 egg whites
1 ⅓ cups apple juice concentrate
½ cup Non-Fat Yogurt (see chapter on Basics)
2 teaspoons vanilla
3 tablespoons cinnamon
1 teaspoon coriander

3 cups whole wheat pastry flour
1 tablespoon baking powder
2 teaspoons baking soda

1 ½ cups Grape-Nuts cereal
6 large Delicious apples unpeeled, sliced by hand or food processor, (8 cups sliced apples)
1 cup chopped walnuts (optional)
¼ cup Cooked Orange Peel (see chapter on Basics), (or 1 tablespoon grated orange rind)

½ cup Grape-Nuts for bottom of pan
½ cup walnut chunks for top, optional

Whisk the first 6 ingredients in a large mixing bowl. Mix together flour, baking powder and soda, and add, all at once, whisking just until blended. Stir in cereal, then fold in sliced apples, nuts and orange peel.

Sprinkle ½ cup of cereal on bottom of a 10-inch tube pan and spread batter evenly over crumbs. Sprinkle walnut chunks on top and press them lightly into batter.

Bake cake in a 350° oven for 1 ½ hours or until cake is dark brown. Serves 10 to 12.

Carob-Honey Cake

This rich moist cake is sure to get raves. It's one of our very favorites.

1 ¼ cups boiling water
¾ cup carob powder

6 egg whites
¾ cup honey
¾ teaspoon dark molasses
1 teaspoon cinnamon
1 cup buttermilk (or ½ cup non-fat yogurt plus ½ cup evaporated skimmed milk)
2 teaspoons vanilla
1 tablespoon oil

1 tablespoon soda
2 cups whole wheat pastry flour

1 cup chopped walnuts (optional)

Whisk hot water and carob powder in a large mixing bowl until smooth then whisk in next 7 ingredients. Mix together flour and soda and whisk in until blended. Fold in nuts if desired.

Spread batter in a 9x13-inch non-stick baking pan, and bake in a 350° oven for approximately 25 to 30 minutes or just until cake tester comes out clean. Do not overbake. This cake should be moist. Serves 10 to 12.

Fluffy Carob Frosting:
¼ cup water
⅓ cup honey

4 egg whites
6 tablespoons carob powder
½ teaspoon coriander
2 teaspoons rum or vanilla

In a 1 ½-quart non-stick saucepan, cook water and honey until boiling rapidly and bubbling for 5 minutes. Meanwhile, in the bowl of an electric mixer, beat egg whites until foamy. Continue beating, slowly adding the honey mixture until whites are stiff and stand in soft peaks. Beat in carob powder, coriander and flavoring until blended. Yields enough frosting for top and sides of one 9x13-inch Carob Honey Cake.

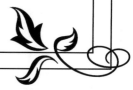

Honey-Bunny Carrot Cake

It is hard to imagine how a cake this rich, moist and delicious can have no yolks and only 1 tablespoon of oil. By eliminating 1 cup of oil in a recipe you can save yourself 1,600 calories.

8 egg whites
1 cup honey
½ cup concentrated apple juice
½ cup water
1 tablespoon oil
1 tablespoon cinnamon
1 tablespoon nutmeg
2 teaspoons vanilla

2 cups whole wheat pastry flour
1 tablespoon baking soda
1 teaspoon baking powder

3 cups grated carrots
½ cup chopped walnuts (optional)
½ cup raisins

Whisk first 8 ingredients in a large mixing bowl. Mix together flour, soda and baking powder and add, all at once, whisking just until blended. Do not overmix. Fold in carrots, nuts and raisins and spread mixture in a non-stick 10-inch tube pan. Bake in a 350° oven for approximately 60 to 65 minutes or just until cake tester comes out clean. Do not overbake. Serves 10 to 12.

Creamy Cheese Walnut Frosting:
2 tablespoons potato starch or cornstarch
2 tablespoons non-fat milk
4 egg whites
½ cup honey

Continues on the next page

2 cups low-fat cottage cheese, whipped

2 tablespoons non-fat yogurt

½ teaspoon ground nutmeg

½ teaspoon ground coriander

1 teaspoon vanilla

1 cup chopped, toasted walnuts

Mix together potato starch or cornstarch with milk and set aside. Beat egg white and honey with electric beater in double boiler over rapidly boiling water for 7 minutes. Beat in cottage cheese, yogurt, spices, vanilla and potato starch mixture; beat with electric beaters until smooth and thick. Stir in half of the chopped nuts. Frost cake and sprinkle remaining nuts on top. Refrigerate cake until serving. This is the perfect frosting for Honey Bunny Carrot Cake. Yields 3 cups frosting.

Old World Plum Custard Cake

This delicious cake was inspired by a plum custard cake our sister-in-law, Dodo, makes. She is a fabulous baker. Ours is without the butter, egg yolks, cream and sugar, and we use whole wheat flour, of course.

Fruit Layer:

12 plums, pitted and cut in half (or 6 peaches, pitted and cut into thick slices)

¼ cup honey

2 teaspoons cinnamon

¼ teaspoon nutmeg

¼ teaspoon coriander

Cake Batter:

½ cup honey

2 egg whites

¾ cup evaporated skimmed milk

½ teaspoon cardamom

½ teaspoon coriander

Continues on the next page

1 ½ cups whole wheat flour
2 teaspoons baking powder

Custard Topping:
3 egg whites
1 ½ cups evaporated skimmed milk
3 tablespoons honey
1 ½ teaspoons whole wheat pastry flour
½ teaspoon vanilla

To prepare fruit layer: Combine fruit and spices and set aside.

To prepare cake batter: Whisk the first 5 ingredients together in a mixing bowl. Mix together flour and baking powder and add, all at once, whisking just until blended. Do not overbeat. Spread batter evenly in a 9x13-inch non-stick baking pan.

To prepare custard topping: Next whisk all of the custard topping ingredients in a large mixing bowl until well mixed.

To assemble cake: Arrange fruit evenly over the batter and pour the custard over the fruit.

Bake in a 350° oven for 35 to 40 minutes. Serve warm or cold. Serves 10 to 12.

Carob Fruit and Spice Cake

The fruit and spices in this moist carob cake gives it an exciting flavor and aroma.

6 egg whites
1 cup honey
¾ teaspoon dark molasses
1 cup non-fat milk
½ cup Non-Fat Yogurt (see chapter on Basics)
4 teaspoons cinnamon
2 teaspoons ginger
1 teaspoon cloves
2 teaspoons vanilla

Continues on the next page

2 cups whole wheat pastry flour

¾ cup carob powder

1 tablespoon baking soda

1 cup boiling water

½ cup crushed pineapple, drained, or ½ cup chopped frozen pitted cherries

½ cup raisins

½ cup Cooked Orange Peel (see chapter on Basics)

½ cup chopped nuts

Whisk the first 9 ingredients in a large mixing bowl. Mix together flour, soda and carob powder and add, all at once, whisking just until blended. Do not overbeat. Mix in boiling water; then stir in nuts and fruits.

Bake cake in a 350° oven for approximately 55 minutes in a 9x13-inch non-stick baking pan. The cake is done when a cake tester comes out clean. Do not overbake. Serves 10 to 12.

Honey Holiday Health Fruit Cake

This delicious and beautiful cake makes a perfect gift to give loved ones and friends around the holiday season. Not only is it a healthy treat but it is also easy to prepare and inexpensive.

1 cup honey

2 cups water

1 pound (or 15-ounce box) black raisins

2 egg whites

½ teaspoon coriander

2 teaspoons nutmeg

3 teaspoons cinnamon

1 cup walnuts or pecans

1 cup Cooked Orange Peel (see chapter on Basics)

2 teaspoons baking soda

2 ¾ cups whole wheat pastry flour

Continues on the next page

Bring the honey, water and raisins to a boil. Lower the heat and cook for 10 minutes uncovered. In a large bowl beat the egg whites lightly with a whisk. Mix in next 5 ingredients and the raisin-honey mixture. Mix together flour and soda and add, ⅓ at a time, mixing just until blended. Do not overmix. Spread mixture in a 10-inch tube pan and bake in a 325° oven for 1 hour and 15 minutes or until top is light brown and cake tests done. Let cake cool before removing from pan. Serves 10 to 12.

Carob Cake Roll with Cream Filling and Pecans

You will be amazed how gourmet and rich tasting this dessert is. It will be hard for your guests to believe that it has very low fat or cholesterol.

Cake Layer:
10 egg whites

½ cup honey
1 teaspoon vanilla
1 teaspoon dark molasses

5 tablespoons carob powder
3 tablespoons whole wheat pastry flour
1 ½ teaspoons Postum (plain, not coffee-flavored)

½ cup chopped pecans, to sprinkle over top of frosted cake

In an electric mixer beat egg whites until foamy. Gradually beat in the honey, vanilla, and molasses until whites are stiff but not dry. Reduce speed and fold in carob, postum and flour. Spread batter evenly on a parchment lined non-stick 10x15-inch jelly roll pan, and bake in a 375° oven for 20 minutes or until lightly browned. Invert cake onto a slightly damp cloth and peel off parchment.

Carob Cream Filling:

1 ⅓ cups evaporated skimmed milk
⅔ cup water
½ cup carob powder
¼ cup whole wheat pastry flour
4 egg whites, slightly beaten
1 ½ teaspoons dry Postum (plain, not coffee-flavored)
⅓ cup honey
1 teaspoon dark molasses

1 teaspoon vanilla
1 teaspoon rum extract (optional)

In a large mixing bowl whisk the first 8 ingredients together. Pour mixture into the top of a double boiler. Heat mixture over medium heat, stirring frequently. Once mixture begins to thicken, stir constantly. Add vanilla and rum extract the last few minutes. Do not allow mixture to boil. Blend until very smooth in a blender or food processor.

To assemble: Reserve a little filling to frost top of cake. Spread remaining filling over entire cake, carefully roll cake up, frost with reserved filling and sprinkle pecans over top. Refrigerate until serving time. Serves 8 to 10.

Carob Angel Cake Filled with Carob Postum Custard

It is hard to imagine that this divine dessert has no cholesterol. It tastes devilishly good.

Carob Angel Cake:
1 ½ cups egg whites (11 or 12 whites)
1 ½ teaspoons cream of tartar
¾ cup honey
½ teaspoon dark molasses
1 teaspoon vanilla

Continues on the next page

¼ cup carob powder

½ cup whole wheat pastry flour

¼ cup potato starch or cornstarch

Beat egg whites in an electric mixer until foamy. Add cream of tartar and gradually beat in honey, molasses and vanilla until whites form soft peaks. Turn beaters to lowest speed and gently fold in carob powder, flour and starch.

Gently spread cake batter evenly in an ungreased 10-inch tube pan. Bake in a 375° oven, with rack set at the bottom position, for 30 to 35 minutes or until cake tests done. Invert cake pan immediately until cool. While it is cooling, prepare the Carob Custard.

Carob-Postum Custard:

6 egg whites

½ cup honey

½ teaspoon dark molasses

¼ cup whole wheat pastry flour

2 cups evaporated skimmed milk

1 teaspoon vanilla

¼ teaspoon cinnamon

6 tablespoons carob powder

4 teaspoons Postum (plain, not coffee-flavored)

2 cups boiling water

Whisk first 7 ingredients in a large mixing bowl. Dissolve carob powder and Postum in the boiling water, add it gradually to egg white mixture and beat well. Pour into an oven proof bowl or souffle dish. Cover and set into a larger pan with enough boiling water to come halfway up the sides of the bowl. Bake custard in a 325° oven until it is set, for approximately 1 ½ hours. Remove from oven, uncover custard and let it cool. Blend until smooth.

To assemble: When frozen, split cake into 3 layers. Return bottom third to tube pan, spread one-third custard over layer. Cover with cake layer and repeat ending with custard on top. Sprinkle top with sliced almonds if desired. Serves 8 to 10.

Note: – *This cake and custard take a lot of baking and cooling time but are well worth it. The entire recipe can be made the day ahead and stored in the refrigerator until serving time.*

– *Be sure to use a tube pan that has inversion legs. Do not attempt to slice cake into layers until cake is frozen.*

Continues on the next page

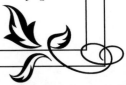

- *If desired drizzle 1 tablespoon of rum over each cake layer before spreading on the custard.*

- *This cake is very soft and creamy, and it should be cut in the kitchen, and served on individual plates.*

Healthy Banana Cake

This moist and delicious health cake can be assembled in minutes. It is a treat you can feel good about serving to family and friends.

1 ½ cups mashed bananas
⅔ cup honey
1 tablespoon oil
6 egg whites
1 teaspoon cinnamon
½ teaspoon coriander
½ teaspoon nutmeg
2 tablespoons buttermilk, or Non-fat Yogurt (see chapter on Basics)
1 ½ teaspoons vanilla
½ cup chopped nuts (optional)

2 ¼ cups whole wheat pastry flour
1 tablespoon baking soda
1 teaspoon baking powder

sprinkle of cinnamon

Whisk first 10 ingredients in a large mixing bowl. Mix together flour, soda and baking powder and add, all at once, whisking just until blended. Do not overmix. Spread evenly in a 9x13-inch non-stick baking pan. Sprinkle cinnamon on top and bake in a 350° oven for 25 minutes or just until a cake tester, inserted in center, comes out clean. Do not overbake. Serves 12.

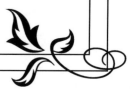

Almond Cake Roll with Italian Cream Filling and Cherries

You are sure to get raves on this one. This dessert can be made the day before.

Cake Layer:
10 egg whites, at room temperature
½ cup honey
1 teaspoon vanilla
1 teaspoon almond extract

6 tablespoons whole wheat pastry flour

Italian Cream Filling:
⅓ cup honey
3 tablespoons potato starch or cornstarch
2 ½ cups evaporated skimmed milk
4 egg whites

1 teaspoon vanilla

Additional Ingredients:
2 cups frozen dark sweet pitted cherries, unsweetened and thawed. Reserve juice.
2 tablespoons Amaretto Liqueur or rum (optional)
1 cup sliced raw almonds, toasted in 400° oven for 7 to 8 minutes, or 1 cup toasted coconut

To prepare cake: In an electric mixer, beat egg whites until foamy. Gradually beat in the honey and extracts until whites are stiff, but not dry. Lower speed and beat in the flour. Carefully spread the batter evenly over a parchment-lined, 10x15-inch jelly roll pan and bake in a 375° oven for approximately 20 minutes or until the cake is lightly browned. Invert cake onto a slightly damp cloth and peel off the parchment.

    To prepare filling: Whisk together all the ingredients (except vanilla) in a mixing bowl, until smooth. Pour mixture into the top of a double boiler, and cook, over simmering water, stirring constantly, until mixture thickens. Stir in vanilla and allow to cool. (If filling happens to get lumpy, puree in a blender or food processor until smooth.)

    To assemble: Arrange the cherries with juice evenly over the cake and drizzle the liqueur over the top. Reserve a little cream filling to frost the top of the cake roll. Spread remaining custard over the entire cake. Carefully, roll cake up, frost top with reserved cream filling and sprinkle with almonds or coconut. Refrigerate until serving time. Serves 10.

Strawberry Cheesecake

This cheesecake is a winner and you won't feel stuffed after eating it, because it's so low in fat. The cheese filling can all be made in a blender or food processor. In strawberry season stand large fresh strawberries on top of cake. What a beauty this cake is and the taste is divine.

Filling:
8 cups low-fat cottage cheese

1 ½ cups honey
2 teaspoons vanilla
¼ teaspoon almond extract
1 tablespoon lemon juice
grated rind of ½ medium lemon
¼ cup potato starch or cornstarch
¼ cup whole wheat pastry flour
12 egg whites

Whip cottage cheese, in batches, in blender or food processor until very smooth. Pour whipped cheese into a large mixing bowl. Blend remaining filling ingredients for 30 seconds and stir this into cheese mixture.

Pour batter into prepared Grape-Nuts Crust and bake in a 325° oven for 45 to 50 minutes or until cheese filling is set, puffed, and light brown. Remove from oven and cool. Meanwhile prepare strawberry glaze.

Grape-Nuts Crust with Cinnamon and Coriander:
¾ cup Grape-Nuts cereal
2 tablespoons concentrated frozen apple juice
1 teaspoon cinnamon
½ teaspoon coriander

Mix all the ingredients together and pat mixture evenly on the bottom of a 9x13-inch glass oven-proof baking pan. Bake the crust in a 350° oven for 7 minutes.

Continues on the next page

Strawberry Glaze:

1 pound frozen whole strawberries, unsweetened

2 tablespoons cornstarch or potato starch

¼ cup honey or ¼ cup concentrated apple juice

Heat strawberries, honey and cornstarch in a non-stick saucepan and cook until glaze is thick and shiny. Gently spread glaze over cheesecake. Refrigerate cake until serving.

Low-Cal Honey Cheese Cake with Blueberry Glaze Topping

This satisfying, delicious and easy-to-prepare cheesecake is one of our standards and favorites.

4 cups low-fat cottage cheese (2 pounds)

½ cup honey

1 tablespoon whole wheat pastry flour

1 tablespoon lemon juice

1 teaspoon lemon rind

6 drops almond extract

1 teaspoon vanilla

6 egg whites

Whip cottage cheese in blender or food processor until smooth. Blend in next 6 ingredients for a minute longer. Whisk egg whites in a large mixing bowl. Add cheese mixture. Spread cheese mixture over prepared Grape-Nuts Crust and bake in a 325° oven for 25 minutes. Do not bake longer. Cheese filling will set as it cools. Refrigerate until serving. Serve plain, with Blueberry Glaze Topping, or with fresh fruit as desired. Serves 6 to 8.

Grape-Nuts Cereal Crust:

½ cup Grape-Nuts cereal

1 ½ tablespoons frozen concentrated apple juice

½ teaspoon cinnamon

Continues on the next page

Mix together cereal, juice and cinnamon in a 9x9-inch non-stick or glass oven-proof baking pan, pat evenly on bottom and bake in 325° oven for 7 minutes.

Blueberry Glaze Topping:
1 10-ounce package frozen blueberries
1 tablespoon cornstarch or potato starch
¼ cup concentrated apple juice
¼ cup water
¼ teaspoon coriander

Heat all ingredients in a non-stick saucepan, stirring constantly until mixture thickens and becomes clear. Stir slowly so that berries will remain whole. While still warm spread carefully on top of cheesecake.

Tall and Fluffy Cheesecake

This fluffy, light, delicious cheesecake was inspired by mama's famous cheesecake. We left out the cream cheese, butter, sour cream and sugar though. You won't miss it. It's marvelous.

Cheese Filling:
5 cups low-fat cottage cheese, whipped
3 tablespoons whole wheat pastry flour
3 tablespoons potato starch or cornstarch
2 teaspoons vanilla
¼ teaspoon almond extract
rind of ½ lemon
1 tablespoon lemon juice
1 teaspoon coriander

10 egg whites (1 ½ cups)
1 cup honey

Whisk first 8 ingredients well in a large mixing bowl. Beat egg whites in an electric mixer until foamy. Gradually beat in honey and continue beating until whites are stiff and shiny. Gently fold egg whites into the cheese mixture and spread filling into prepared Grape-Nuts Crust.

Continues on the next page

Bake cheesecake in a 350° oven for 50 minutes, then turn off heat and let cake remain in oven until cool with oven door closed. Refrigerate until serving. Serves 8 to 10.

Grape-Nuts-Pecan Crust:
¾ cup Grape-Nuts cereal
½ cup chopped pecans
2 tablespoons concentrated apple juice
½ teaspoon cinnamon

Mix all the ingredients together and pat mixture evenly on the bottom of a 10-inch spring form. Bake crust in a 350° oven for 7 minutes.

Party Apple Casserole

This dessert is great for parties and can be prepared quickly without peeling the apples or making a crust. Serve warm or cold.

1 cup Grape-Nuts cereal for crust

16 cups thinly sliced Delicious apples (approximately 12 large apples), skin left on (apples may be sliced in food processor)
2 tablespoons cinnamon
1 cup concentrated frozen apple juice
½ teaspoon coriander

½ cup Grape-Nuts cereal for topping
½ cup chopped walnuts or pecans
1 teaspoon cinnamon
2 tablespoons concentrated apple juice

sprinkle of cinnamon for top

Sprinkle 1 cup of Grape-Nuts cereal evenly on the bottom of a 9x13-inch glass oven-proof or non-stick baking dish. Toss next 4 ingredients in a large mixing bowl. Spread apple slices evenly over cereal and pour juice left in the bowl over apple slices.

Mix together next 4 ingredients for topping. Sprinkle topping evenly over the apple slices and sprinkle cinnamon generously on top. Cover with foil and pierce foil in several places with a sharp knife to allow steam to escape.

Bake in a 400° oven for 1 hour or until apple slices are tender. Remove foil and allow casserole to brown for 10 to 15 minutes. Serves 10 to 12.

Oatmeal-Raisin Chews

These easy-to-prepare, healthy chews are sweetened primarily with apple juice. They're great for snacks. We enjoy these frozen.

2 cups rolled oats, toasted for 8 to 10 minutes in 350° oven
2 teaspoons cinnamon
2 teaspoons nutmeg
1 teaspoon coriander
¼ cup shredded coconut
¼ cup black raisins
¼ cup chopped nuts (optional)
½ cup frozen concentrated apple juice

4 egg whites

2 teaspoons honey

Mix together first 8 ingredients in a large mixing bowl. Beat egg whites in an electric mixer until foamy. Beat in honey until stiff but not dry, then gently fold egg whites into cereal mixture. Immediately drop by teaspoon onto two non-stick cookie sheets and bake in 425° oven for 20 minutes or until they are dark brown. Yields 36 to 48 cookies.

Carrot Dessert Squares

What could be better than this moist, flavorful, satisfying, healthy treat?

¼ cup concentrated frozen apple juice
¼ cup water
½ cup honey
1 tablespoon oil
4 egg whites
1 teaspoon vanilla
1 ½ teaspoons nutmeg
1 ½ teaspoons cinnamon

1 teaspoon soda
1 cup whole wheat pastry flour

1 ½ cups grated carrots
½ cup black raisins
½ cup chopped walnuts (optional)

Whisk first 8 ingredients in large bowl. Mix together flour and soda, and add, all at once, whisking just until smooth. Fold in carrots, raisins and nuts. Bake in a 9x9-inch non-stick baking pan at 350° for 45 minutes.

This recipe can be doubled and baked in a 9x13-inch non-stick baking pan for approximately 55 to 60 minutes or just until cake tester comes out clean. This cake should be moist. Do not overbake. Cool and cut into squares. Serves 6 to 9.

Raisin Sweetened Carob Brownies

These brownies are so healthy and so yummy. They won't last.

¾ cup carob powder
1 cup boiling water

Continues on the next page

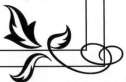

6 egg whites
1 cup raisins

1 cup evaporated skimmed milk
½ cup Non-Fat Yogurt (see chapter on Basics)
4 tablespoons honey
¾ teaspoon dark molasses
1 tablespoon oil
1 tablespoon vanilla

1 tablespoon baking soda
2 cups whole wheat pastry flour

1 cup chopped walnuts (optional)

Whisk carob powder and boiling water in a large mixing bowl until smooth. Chop raisins in blender with egg whites and add this to carob mixture. Whisk in next 6 ingredients until smooth, then mix together flour and soda and add, all at once, whisking just until blended. Do not overmix. Fold in nuts. Spread evenly in a 9x13-inch non-stick baking pan and bake in a 350° oven for 25 to 30 minutes or just until cake tester comes out clean. Do not overbake. Serves 10 to 12.

Coconut Haystacks (GF)

Here are delicious and healthy coconut haystacks you can feel good about eating and serving.

4 egg whites

½ cup honey
1 teaspoon vanilla

½ cup chopped walnuts
½ cup crushed date pieces or chunks
4 cups shredded, unsweetened, coconut (or 2 cups coconut and 2 cups cereal flakes)

Beat egg whites with electric mixer on high speed until foamy. Gradually beat in honey and vanilla and continue beating until whites are thick and shiny. Fold in nuts, dates and coconuts by hand and drop by heaping teaspoon onto non-stick cookie sheets. Bake in a 350° oven for approximately 20 minutes or until golden brown and dry on the outside. Yields 36 to 40.

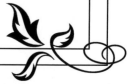

Crispy Carob Cookies

It's so great to be able to eat crispy carob cookies and to know they're made with only healthy, pure ingredients, without fat or cholesterol.

4 cups whole wheat flakes cereal (made without sugar and without salt if possible)

4 egg whites

⅓ cup honey
¼ teaspoon dark molasses
1 teaspoon vanilla
½ cup carob powder

Place cereal in a large mixing bowl. In an electric mixer in separate bowl beat egg whites until foamy. Gradually beat in honey, molasses, vanilla, and carob powder and continue beating until whites are stiff and glossy. Quickly fold egg white mixture into cereal, and immediately drop by rounded teaspoon onto two non-stick cookie sheets. Bake in a 400° oven for 15 to 20 minutes. Yields 36 to 48 cookies.

Light Date-Nut Cookies

These beautiful, light and healthy cookies are especially delicious.

1 cup pecans

1 cup dates (or ½ cup dates and ½ cup raisins)
2 egg whites, unbeaten

4 egg whites, beaten

2 tablespoons honey
1 teaspoon vanilla

1 teaspoon cinnamon
½ cup whole wheat flour
½ teaspoon baking powder

Continues on the next page

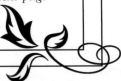

Chop pecans in a blender or food processor. Blend in dates and 2 egg whites until dates are well mashed. Place date mixture in a large mixing bowl and set aside.

Beat 4 egg whites in an electric mixer until foamy. Gradually beat in honey and vanilla and continue beating until whites are thick and shiny. Mix together cinnamon, flour and baking powder. Reduce speed and lightly fold dry ingredients into whites. Stir ½ of the egg white mixture into the date mixture, then carefully fold in the remaining egg white mixture.

Drop by spoonfuls onto two non-stick cookie sheets and bake in a 350° oven for approximately 20 minutes or until light brown. Yields 30 to 36 cookies.

Spicy Raisin Balls

These attractive cookies have a great flavor and texture. Since these are sweetened only with fruit, you can eat them without guilt.

1 cup raisins
¼ cup concentrated frozen apple juice (or ¾ cup of unsweetened apple juice, omit water)
½ cup water

1 egg white
2 tablespoons Homemade Non-Fat Yogurt or commercial brand, (see chapter on Basics)

1 cup whole wheat flour
½ teaspoon baking soda
2 teaspoons cinnamon
¼ teaspoon nutmeg
¼ teaspoon ground cloves

¼ cup chopped nuts (optional)

½ cup chopped nuts (or ½ cup Grape-Nuts cereal) for coating balls

In a non-stick saucepan bring raisins, apple juice and water to a boil. Cool mixture slightly in a mixing bowl, then stir in the egg white and yogurt. Mix together flour, baking soda and spices. Stir into raisin mixture, then fold in ¼ cup of nuts.

Form the dough into small round balls with damp hands. Coat each ball with chopped nuts or cereal and arrange balls on a non-stick cookie sheet. Bake in a 350° oven for approximately 20 minutes or until cookies are golden brown. Yields 18 cookies.

Carrot and Raisin Chews

These are such favorites that we keep a 5-pound honey can full in the freezer for satisfying healthy snacks. We enjoy them best frozen.

½ cup honey
½ cup concentrated apple juice
4 egg whites
1 teaspoon vanilla

4 teaspoons cinnamon
1 teaspoon nutmeg
¼ teaspoon cloves
1 teaspoon baking powder
1 cup whole wheat flour

2 ½ cups rolled oats, uncooked
2 cups grated carrots
¾ cup black raisins
¾ cup chopped nuts (optional)

1 cup Grape-Nuts cereal
1 teaspoon cinnamon

Whisk first 4 ingredients in a large mixing bowl until well blended. Mix together spices, flour and baking powder, and add, all at once, whisking just until blended. Fold in oats, carrots, raisins and nuts. Drop by rounded teaspoon one at a time into a mixture of cereal and cinnamon. Coat well with cereal, arrange cookies on a non-stick cookie sheet, and flatten cookies down with a fork. Bake in a 350° oven for approximately 20 to 30 minutes, or until dark brown. Yields 36 to 48 cookies.

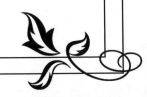

Munchy Mandelbrot (Almond Cookies)

If you like crunchy snacks, you'll enjoy these. They are made with only the healthiest ingredients.

6 egg whites
1 cup honey
1 teaspoon vanilla
½ teaspoon allspice
2 teaspoons cinnamon
½ teaspoon cloves

3 cups whole wheat flour
2 teaspoons baking powder

1 cup chopped almonds (or sliced, or slivered almonds)
1 cup raisins
¼ cup chopped, Cooked Orange Peel (see chapter on Basics)

sprinkle of cinnamon for top

Whisk the first 6 ingredients in a mixing bowl. Mix together flour and baking powder and add, all at once, whisking just until blended. Then stir in almonds, raisins and orange peel. For easy shaping of loaves, chill dough overnight or for several hours. Preheat oven to 350°. Shape into 8 small loaves, 4x2x1-inch, each. Bake on a non-stick cookie sheet in a 350° oven for approximately 30 minutes or until loaves are lightly brown. Remove loaves from oven.

Cut loaves into slices ½-inch thick. Arrange slices on two non-stick cookie sheets. Sprinkle slices with cinnamon and bake for 1 hour in a 225° oven or until slices are dry and crispy. Yields approximately 5 dozen Mandelbrot cookies.

Date-Carob Brownies

The taste of these moist, healthy brownies is a true delight.

¾ cup non-fat milk
¼ cup Non-Fat Yogurt (see chapter on Basics)
6 egg whites
⅓ cup honey
2 teaspoons vanilla
1 tablespoon oil
¾ teaspoon dark molasses

2 cups whole wheat pastry flour
2 teaspoons baking soda

¾ cup carob powder
1 ½ cups boiling water

½ pound (⅔ cup) mashed dates
½ cup chopped walnuts (optional)

In a large mixing bowl whisk the first 7 ingredients. Mix together flour and baking soda and add, all at once, whisking just until smooth. Mix carob powder with boiling water and whisk it into flour mixture. Stir in dates and optional walnuts. Spread batter in a 9x13-inch non-stick baking pan and bake in a 350° oven for 25 minutes or just until cake tester comes out clean. These brownies are best moist. Do not overbake. Serves 10 to 12.

Note: — *1 cup of buttermilk can be substituted for the non-fat milk and yogurt in this recipe. Honey can be eliminated by adding ⅓ cup additional mashed dates.*

Pumpkin Cereal Spice Chews

It is so satisfying to munch on these healthy chews. Your family and friends will love them.

1 ½ cups pumpkin puree
4 egg whites
⅔ cup honey
1 teaspoon vanilla

1 cup whole wheat flour
1 teaspoon baking powder
1 tablespoon cinnamon
1 teaspoon nutmeg
1 teaspoon ginger
1 teaspoon coriander
¼ teaspoon ground cloves

1 cup oats
1 cup cracked wheat
½ cup bran
1 cup black raisins

1 ½ cups Grape Nuts cereal
1 ½ teaspoons cinnamon

In a large mixing bowl whisk first 4 ingredients until frothy. Mix together flour, baking powder and spices, and add all at once, whisking just until smooth. Stir in oats, cracked wheat, bran and raisins.

In a small bowl mix together Grape-Nuts cereal and cinnamon. Drop cookie dough into cereal by spoonfuls, and arrange cookies on 2 non-stick cookie sheets. Flatten cookies by pressing them with a fork. Bake in a 350-degree oven for 25 to 30 minutes or until cookies are browned. Yields 36 to 48 cookies.

Spicy Pumpkin Cereal Bars

These healthy, delicious treats are made with whole wheat flour and are spicy and wonderful. Who needs rich, sugary sweets, when these taste so good. These are delicious frozen.

1 cup Grape-Nuts cereal
1 ½ teaspoons cinnamon
1 ½ cups canned pumpkin puree
1 cup honey
6 egg whites
1 tablespoon cinnamon
1 teaspoon each, ginger, nutmeg and coriander
¼ teaspoon ground cloves

1 cup whole wheat flour
1 teaspoon baking soda
1 teaspoon baking powder

2 cups rolled oats
1 cup raisins
1 cup chopped walnuts (optional)

Mix together cinnamon and Grape-Nuts cereal. Spread this mixture evenly on the bottom of a 10x15-inch non-stick jelly roll pan. In a large bowl beat together the pumpkin, honey, egg whites, and spices. Mix together the flour, baking soda and baking powder. Add this, beating just until blended. Stir in oats, raisins and walnuts.

To spread the pumpkin mixture on top of the Grape-Nuts in the jelly roll pan, drop batter by tablespoonful on top of the cereal; then spread gently to cover entire pan. Bake in a 350-degree oven for 35 to 40 minutes or until top is firm to the touch and light brown in color. Allow to cool, then cut into squares with a plastic spatula. Store in refrigerator or freezer. Yields 36 to 48 bars.

Date-Raisin-Oat-Bran Balls

These healthy, fruit sweetened cookies are great tasting.

½ cup pitted dates
½ cup raisins
2 egg whites

¼ cup non-fat milk
1 tablespoon honey
1 teaspoon vanilla
1 teaspoon cinnamon

2 cups rolled oats, toasted in a 400° oven on a non-stick cookie sheet for 8 to 10
    minutes or until lightly brown
¼ cup bran

Mash dates, raisins and egg whites in a blender or food processor. Place this mixture into a mixing bowl. Stir in next 4 ingredients and mix well, then stir in oats and bran. Form into small balls the size of walnuts with moistened hands. Place balls on non-stick cookie sheet. They can be placed close together since they do not rise. Sprinkle with cinnamon and bake in a 400° oven for 10 to 15 minutes or until brown. Recipe makes approximately 50 balls.

Mixture can also be made into bars instead of balls by baking the oat-date mixture in a 9x13-inch non-stick baking pan. Sprinkle lightly with cinnamon and bake in 400° oven until dark brown, for approximately 12 to 15 minutes. Cool slightly and cut into bars. Yields 18 cookies.

Puffed Wheat Crisps

These are for folks who enjoy crispy, healthy treats. They can be prepared quickly and stored in an airtight container or in the freezer. They may be eaten frozen.

Continues on the next page

½ cup honey

2 tablespoons water

¼ teaspoon ginger

½ teaspoon cinnamon

6 cups puffed wheat cereal (without salt, sugar or oil)

Boil honey, water and spices in a large non-stick saucepan until it foams and rises. This will take only a few minutes. Quickly stir in puffed wheat cereal. When cereal is coated pour mixture into a 9x13-inch non-stick pan and bake in a 350° oven for 15 minutes or until lightly brown and crispy. Remove from oven and press down slightly with spatula. When cool break into pieces. Yields 12 to 15 pieces.

Cooked Honey Oatmeal Cookies

These great cookies are easy and fun to make, and so healthy and chewy to eat.

⅔ cup rolled oats

¼ cup whole wheat flour

⅔ cup evaporated skimmed milk

½ cup honey

1 teaspoon cinnamon

¼ teaspoon ginger

¼ teaspoon cloves

½ cup Grape-Nuts cereal

½ teaspoon cinnamon

Mix together first 7 ingredients in a non-stick frying pan. Cook over medium heat until mixture bubbles, stirring frequently. Remove from heat.

Mix Grape-Nuts cereal and ½ teaspoon cinnamon into a small bowl. Drop one rounded teaspoon of cookie mixture into cereal. Coat each cookie lightly with cereal and arrange them on a non-stick cookie sheet. Flatten each cookie down with a fork. Bake in a 375° oven for 20 minutes or until dark brown. Yields 18 cookies.

Tofu Custard

This is a simple, healthy, and delicious dessert.

16 ounces tofu (the softest and smoothest you can find)
½ cup honey
1 tablespoon whole wheat pastry flour
⅛ teaspoon cardamom
⅛ teaspoon coriander
1 teaspoon vanilla
2 teaspoons lemon juice
¼ teaspoon nutmeg, sprinkled on top

6 egg whites

sprinkle of nutmeg for top

Blend first 8 ingredients in a blender or food processor (or beat in an electric mixer until smooth). Add egg whites and beat for a moment longer. Pour tofu mixture into a 9-inch glass oven-proof pie plate. Sprinkle nutmeg on top and bake in a 325° oven for 25 minutes. Do not bake longer. Custard will set when chilled. Serves 6.

Brandied Poached Pear Halves (GF)

This simple and delicious dessert is sweetened entirely with fruit juice.

4 large winter pears, peeled and cut in half, cored
½ cup concentrated apple juice
2 teaspoons cinnamon
¼ teaspoon coriander

1 tablespoon brandy (optional)

Continues on the next page

Simmer pear halves in apple juice and spices in a large non-stick pan turning pears at least once. Cook only until tender when pierced with a fork. Add brandy and store in refrigerator. Serves 6 to 8.

Spicy Baked Apples (GF)

The aroma of these apples baking is a real treat. We enjoy them for breakfast, dessert or snacks. They are healthy and so easy to prepare.

4 large Roman Beauty apples, cores removed, leaving a ½-inch base

1 teaspoon cinnamon
4 whole cloves
sprinkle of nutmeg
8 teaspoons concentrated apple juice

1 cup water
1 teaspoon cinnamon
2 cloves

Place cored apples in a 9-inch glass oven-proof pie plate. Fill each apple with ¼ teaspoon cinnamon, one clove, a dash of nutmeg and 2 teaspoons concentrated apple juice. Pour water around apples and add spices. Bake in 350° oven for approximately 1 ½ hours or until apples are brown and soft to touch. Remove from oven and baste with its own juice. Store in refrigerator. Serves 4.

Pears Poached with Coriander and Cardamom with Honey Vanilla Sauce (GF)

This delicious, rich tasting dessert is very low in calories and has no fat or cholesterol. For a luscious dessert spoon Honey Vanilla Sauce over each pear half and top with a sprinkle of coriander.

Continues on the next page

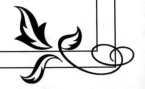

3 large green winter pears (firm and nearly ripe), halved, cored, and peeled

⅓ cup concentrated frozen apple juice
¾ teaspoon coriander
¾ teaspoon cardamom

sprinkle of coriander for top

Arrange pear halves core side down in a large pot or large covered frying pan. Pour juice and spices over the pears. Simmer the pears over low heat for 10 minutes then turn pear halves over and simmer an additional 10 to 15 minutes, or until pears are barely tender when pierced with a fork. Remove pear halves gently from pan, place pears in a bowl, pour juice over them, and chill. Serve pear halves with a sprinkle of coriander. Serves 4 to 6.

Honey Vanilla Sauce (GF)

This sauce is delicious over Spicy Baked Apples, Apple Crepes, slices of Giant Apple Cake and over Yummy Yam Souffle too! It keeps well in the refrigerator for a week.

4 egg whites
¼ cup honey
1 teaspoon vanilla extract
⅓ cup evaporated skimmed milk

Heat all the ingredients in the top of a double boiler over gently simmering water. Use a whisk to beat mixture until it thickens. Sauce will thicken quickly once the water below is boiling. Do not allow sauce to boil. When sauce has thickened, if the consistency is not smooth, puree sauce in blender or food processor until smooth Refrigerate until serving.

Dark Moist Bran Muffins

These dark, moist muffins taste almost like cake and they're so good for you.

1 cup evaporated skimmed milk (or 1 ½ cups non-fat milk and omit water)
½ cup water
½ cup Homemade Non-Fat Yogurt (see chapter on Basics), or commercial brand
½ cup honey
2 tablespoons dark molasses
2 egg whites

2 cups whole wheat flour plus 1 tablespoon flour
1 ½ teaspoons baking soda

1 ½ cups bran flakes

Whisk the first 6 ingredients in a large mixing bowl. Mix together flour and soda, and add, whisking just until smooth. Do not overmix. Stir in bran. Fill non-stick muffin cups to the top and bake in a 350° oven for 20 to 25 minutes. Remove gently from muffin cups. Yields 12.

Quick Apple Pie

This healthy and delicious pie takes only minutes to assemble. A friend of ours has been making her husband this pie daily for years, ever since they both tasted it at our home. Serve warm or cold.

½ cup Grape-Nuts cereal

6 large Delicious apples, unpeeled, sliced thin (may be sliced in food processor)
⅓ cup concentrated apple juice
½ teaspoon coriander
1 tablespoon cinnamon
sprinkle of cinnamon for top

Continues on the next page

Sprinkle Grape-Nuts on the bottom of a 9-inch glass oven-proof pie plate. Mix together next 4 ingredients in a large bowl. Spread apple mixture over cereal in pie plate and pour juice left in bowl over the apple slices. Sprinkle with cinnamon. Cover pie tightly with foil. Pierce foil with a sharp knife in several places to allow steam to escape and bake in a 400° oven for approximately 40 to 45 minutes or until apples are tender. Remove foil and allow pie to brown for 10 to 15 minutes longer. Serves 6.

Pineapple Cheese Pie

This pie is simple to make, healthy to serve and delicious to eat. What more can one ask for?

3 cups low-fat cottage cheese

⅓ cup honey
1 tablespoon whole wheat pastry flour
1 teaspoon lemon juice
¼ teaspoon almond extract
½ teaspoon vanilla

5 egg whites

1 cup crushed pineapple, well drained
¼ teaspoon coriander

Whip cottage cheese in a blender or food processor until smooth. Blend in next 5 ingredients for 30 seconds longer. In a large bowl beat egg whites with a whisk. Stir in cottage cheese mixture.

To assemble: Spread pineapple mixed with coriander evenly over prepared Grape-Nuts Crust, then pour cheese filling over pineapple. Bake pie in a 325° oven for 25 minutes. Do not bake longer. Cheese filling will set as it chills. Serves 6.

Grape-Nuts-Coconut Crust:
½ cup Grape-Nuts cereal
1 ½ tablespoons concentrated apple juice
½ teaspoon cinnamon
¼ cup shredded coconut, unsweetened

Mix all ingredients together and pat mixture evenly on the bottom of a 9-inch glass oven-proof pie plate. Bake crust in a 325° oven for 7 minutes.

Blueberry Cheese Pie

For a delicious and easy-to-prepare blueberry cheese pie, follow directions for Pineapple Cheese Pie above, omitting pineapple. After pouring cheese filling into a pie crust, drop 1 cup frozen unthawed or fresh blueberries into pie filling and bake in a 325° oven for 25 minutes. Do not bake longer. Cheese filling will set as it chills. Serves 6.

Tofu-Banana-Pineapple Pie

This is an excellent dessert with a delightful flavor. It is relatively low in calories, too.

2 12-ounce packages of medium firm tofu, rinsed, drained and patted dry
4 egg whites
2 tablespoons whole wheat pastry flour
½ cup honey
2 tablespoons lemon juice
1 teaspoon vanilla
½ teaspoon coriander
2 medium size ripe bananas

1 8-ounce can of crushed pineapple, unsweetened, well drained

Puree first 8 ingredients in blender or food processor. Fold in pineapple and pour mixture into prepared Grape-Nuts Crust. Bake in 325° oven for approximately 25 minutes or until the center jiggles slightly. Cool before refrigerating. Decorate top with fresh fruit. Serves 6.

Grape-Nuts Crust with Cardamom and Coriander:
½ cup Grape-Nuts cereal
1 ½ tablespoons concentrated apple juice
½ teaspoon cardamom
½ teaspoon coriander

Combine ingredients in a 9-inch glass oven-proof plate. Pat evenly on the bottom and partially bake in 325° oven for 7 minutes.

Note: — Do not bake longer than 25 minutes. Custard will set when chilled.

Crustless Pumpkin Pie (GF)

It's so wonderful to be able to enjoy a delicious pumpkin pie without cream, sugar, and egg yolks. This recipe makes 2 pies. We prefer no crust on this one.

8 egg whites
¾ cup honey
2 teaspoons cinnamon
1 teaspoon ginger
½ teaspoon cloves

1 29-ounce can of pumpkin
3 cups evaporated skimmed milk (or 1 ½ cups evaporated skimmed milk and 1 ½ cups
   non-fat milk)
2 ½ tablespoons whole wheat pastry flour or Gluten Free flour

Preheat oven to 425°. Whisk first 5 ingredients in a large mixing bowl until frothy. Whisk in pumpkin, milk and flour until smooth. Pour into two 9-inch glass oven-proof pie plates. **Reduce oven temperature to 350°** and bake for 30 minutes. Do not bake longer. Filling will set as it cools. Serves 8 to 10.

Baked Vanilla Custard Pie (Crustless) (GF)

A custard lover will adore this velvety smooth custard pie, made without the cholesterol found in regular custard pies. You can really enjoy yourself.

1 ⅔ cups evaporated skimmed milk
1 cup non-fat milk
6 egg whites
⅓ cup honey
1 tablespoon whole wheat or Gluten Free flour
1 teaspoon vanilla

¼ teaspoon nutmeg, sprinkled on top

Continues on the next page

Whisk together first 6 ingredients. Pour mixture into a 9-inch glass oven-proof pie plate and sprinkle with nutmeg. Bake for 25 to 30 minutes in 325° oven, or bake in custard cups for 15 to 20 minutes. Do not bake longer. Custard will set as it chills. Serves 4 to 6.

Custard Bread Pudding (GF)

This healthy and delightful bread pudding can be served warm or cold for a breakfast or brunch, or as a dessert. The grain in the bread, with the milk and egg whites, provide a nourishing protein dessert.

8 slices of soft whole wheat or Gluten Free bread

2 ⅔ cups evaporated skimmed milk
6 egg whites
⅓ cup honey
1 teaspoon vanilla
1 teaspoon cinnamon

sprinkle of nutmeg

Line the bottom of a 9x9-inch non-stick or glass oven-proof baking dish with 4 slices of bread. In a large mixing bowl whisk the next 5 ingredients. Pour ½ of the custard mixture over the bread slices in baking pan. Cover with more bread slices and pour the remaining ½ of the custard over these slices. Sprinkle with nutmeg. Bake bread pudding in a 375° oven for 30 to 35 minutes or until custard is set and begins to puff up slightly. Serves 6.

Brown Rice-Raisin Pudding (GF)

This healthy rice pudding has such a delicious flavor. Serve it hot or cold.

4 cups cooked brown rice
6 egg whites
1 cup non-fat milk (or evaporated skimmed milk for richer texture and taste)
½ cup honey
1 tablespoon vanilla
½ teaspoon coriander
1 tablespoon cinnamon

1 cup black raisins

½ cup chopped walnuts for topping (optional)
2 tablespoons honey for topping (optional)

sprinkle of cinnamon for topping

Whisk the first 7 ingredients in a large mixing bowl until well mixed. Stir in raisins. Pour mixture into a 9x13-inch non-stick or glass oven-proof baking pan. Top with nuts and honey. Sprinkle generously with cinnamon and bake in a 375° oven for 30 to 35 minutes. Serves 8 to 10.

Apple-Custard Delight

This recipe is a true delight to look at, to serve, and to eat.

3 cups puffed wheat cereal

8 cups Delicious apples, sliced. (They can be sliced in food processor.)
6 ounces concentrated frozen apple juice
½ teaspoon coriander
2 teaspoons cinnamon

Continues on the next page

1 ⅔ cups evaporated skimmed milk

1 cup non-fat milk

6 egg whites

⅓ cup honey

1 tablespoon whole wheat flour

1 teaspoon vanilla

½ teaspoon coriander

generous sprinkle of nutmeg for top

Sprinkle cereal on bottom of a 9x13-inch non-stick or glass oven-proof baking dish. Mix together apple slices, apple juice and spices in a large mixing bowl. Spread apple mixture over cereal in baking pan and pour apple juice left in bowl over the apple slices. Cover with foil and pierce foil with a sharp knife in 8 to 10 places as you would pierce a pie crust. Bake covered in 400° oven for 25 minutes, then uncovered for 10 minutes.

Meanwhile whisk next 7 ingredients in a large mixing bowl. Remove apple casserole from oven and pour custard over the hot baked apple slices. Top with nutmeg. Reduce oven temperature to 350° and continue baking casserole uncovered for 12 to 15 minutes or until custard is set. Do not bake longer. Custard will set as it chills. Serves 8 to 10.

Pineapple-Lemon Souffle (GF)

This recipe makes a delicious, light, yet filling dessert. The leftovers can be enjoyed cold.

Pineapple-Lemon Sauce:
2 cups unsweetened pineapple juice

2 tablespoons honey

½ teaspoon coriander

1 tablespoon potato or cornstarch

1 tablespoon lemon juice

½ teaspoon lemon rind

½ cup crushed pineapple, drained

Continues on the next page

Slowly heat the first 4 ingredients in a non-stick saucepan until mixture comes to a boil. Allow mixture to simmer for 5 minutes. Stir in lemon juice and rind. Reserve 1 cup of sauce. Pour the remaining sauce on the bottom of a 2-quart souffle dish along with crushed pineapple.

Pineapple-Lemon Meringue:
8 egg whites
¼ cup honey
1 cup Pineapple-Lemon Sauce

Beat egg whites in an electric mixer until foamy. Gradually beat in honey until whites are stiff but not dry. Reduce speed to low and gently fold in reserved sauce. Gently spread egg white mixture into souffle dish over Pineapple-Lemon Sauce. Bake in a 375° oven for 15 minutes or until souffle is puffed and light brown on top and serve immediately. Cut large slices of meringue and spoon sauce on bottom of souffle dish over each serving. Serves 4 to 6.

Fluffy Carob Souffle

It is hard to believe that these wholesome ingredients can be transformed into such a delicious and impressive taste treat. You'll have to experience it yourself to believe it.

Carob Sauce:
1 cup boiling water
2 teaspoons Postum (plain, not coffee-flavored)
¼ cup carob powder

1 ½ cups evaporated skimmed milk
½ teaspoon dark molasses
¼ cup honey
⅛ teaspoon cinnamon

3 tablespoons whole wheat pastry flour

½ teaspoon vanilla
1 to 2 tablespoons rum or Cognac (or 1 teaspoon rum extract), (optional)

Continues on the next page

In a large mixing bowl dissolve the carob powder and Postum in boiling water. Whisk in the milk, honey, molasses and cinnamon, and then flour. Cook sauce in the top of a double boiler until slightly thickened, stirring occasionally with a whisk. Add vanilla and liquor. Reserve 1 cup of sauce for meringue and pour remaining sauce in the bottom of a 2-quart souffle dish or oven-proof bowl.

Carob Meringue:
8 egg whites
¼ cup carob powder
¼ cup honey
½ teaspoon dark molasses
1 cup Carob Sauce
sprinkle of cinnamon

Beat egg whites in an electric mixer until foamy. Gradually beat in carob powder, then honey and molasses until whites are stiff but not dry. Reduce speed to low and gently fold in 1 cup of the hot Carob Sauce. Gently spread the egg white mixture in the prepared souffle dish on top of the Carob Sauce. Bake souffle in a 375° oven for 15 minutes or just until souffle is puffed and light brown. Serve immediately. Cut meringue in slices and spoon sauce from bottom of souffle dish over the meringue with a sprinkle of cinnamon over each portion. Serves 4 to 6.

Soft Meringue Shell Filled with Strawberry Banana Yogurt Topped with Strawberry Sauce (GF)

This spectacular low-calorie dessert is bound to bring oohs and aahs from your guests. The meringue shell and sauce can be done well in advance, and the soft frozen yogurt filling takes only a few minutes to prepare.

Soft Meringue Shell:
8 egg whites
⅓ cup honey
1 teaspoon almond extract
2 tablespoons potato starch or corn starch

Continues on the next page

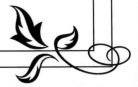

154

Strawberry-Banana Yogurt:

2 cups plain non-fat yogurt, frozen into cubes in ice cube tray, commercial brand or
     homemade (see chapter on Basics)

1 cup frozen strawberries (or frozen blueberries), unthawed

¼ cup frozen concentrated apple juice, unthawed

2 ripe bananas, cut into pieces for blender

¼ teaspoon coriander

Strawberry Sauce:

¼ cup honey (or ¼ cup concentrated apple juice)

2 tablespoons cornstarch or potato starch

½ cup water

¼ teaspoon coriander

2 teaspoons lemon juice

2 cups frozen strawberries, unthawed

To prepare meringue shell: In an electric mixer beat egg whites until foamy. Gradually beat in the honey and almond extract and continue beating until egg whites are thick and glossy. Fold in starch. Gently spread mixture into a 10-inch spring form, hollowing out center and mounding mixture around outer edges to form a shell. Bake at 250° for 1 hour and turn off oven. Allow meringue shell to stay in oven for at least 1 hour or longer before removing. When cool freeze in spring form pan until ready to use.

    To prepare soft frozen yogurt: Approximately 20 to 30 minutes before serving, puree the frozen yogurt cubes and remaining ingredients, in a blender or food processor (in batches if necessary). Spread mixture immediately into the frozen meringue shell and freeze until ready to serve.

    To prepare strawberry sauce: Combine all ingredients in a non-stick saucepan reserving half of strawberries to add later on. Heat to a boiling point and boil gently, stirring constantly for 1 minute. Stir in remaining berries. Chill.

    To assemble: Just before serving remove side from spring form and pile fresh fruit on top. Cut generous slices and top with strawberry sauce. Serves 6 to 8.

Pineapple Creamy Soft Frozen Yogurt (GF)

It is hard to believe that something so easy to prepare and without sugar, fat or cholesterol can be so creamy and delicious.

1 6-ounce can of concentrated frozen pineapple juice
1 cup Non-Fat Yogurt (see chapter on Basics)
1 cup evaporated skimmed milk
½ teaspoon coriander
⅛ teaspoon nutmeg

Blend all ingredients together until foamy. Pour mixture into a 1-quart bowl or container, and place in freezer for 25 to 30 minutes. Serve at once. In case it should freeze, remove it from the freezer ½ hour before serving, and thaw just until it can be cut into chunks with a sharp knife. Whip in blender or food processor until smooth, and serve at once.

Note: — We enjoy this only partially frozen. Then it tastes the creamiest. Serves 2 to 3.

Soft Frozen Blueberry-Banana Yogurt Dessert

2 cups plain Non-Fat Yogurt, frozen (see chapter on Basics) (GF)

2 ripe bananas
1 cup frozen blueberries or 2 cups frozen strawberries
¼ cup frozen concentrated apple juice

Thaw frozen yogurt just long enough to cut it into chunks with sharp knife. Puree chunks of frozen yogurt and remaining ingredients in a blender or food processor. Serve immediately, or freeze for 15 minutes before serving. Serves 4.

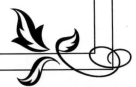

Soft Frozen Grape-Banana Yogurt (GF)

This is great to make in the summer when green grapes are in season. It is very refreshing, healthy and easy to prepare.

1 cup Non-Fat Yogurt (see chapter on Basics)
1 cup frozen seedless green grapes
1 frozen banana

Blend in food processor or blender until smooth. Serve immediately, or chill for 15 minutes before serving. Serves 2 to 3.

Spiced Apple Soft Frozen Yogurt (GF)

You can prepare this healthy dessert in five minutes. It makes 1-quart.

1 6-ounce can concentrated frozen apple juice
½ cup Non-Fat Yogurt (see chapter on Basics)
1 ½ cups evaporated skimmed milk
1 teaspoon cinnamon
½ teaspoon coriander
⅛ teaspoon nutmeg
½ teaspoon vanilla

Blend all ingredients together until foamy. Pour mixture into a 1-quart bowl or container and place in freezer.

Note: – This yogurt tastes best eaten only partially frozen. It gets hard and icy if frozen completely. In case it should freeze, remove it from freezer ½ hour before serving, thaw it slightly, cut it into pieces and blend it in a blender or food processor. Serve immediately. Serves 4.

Easy Fat-Free Soft Orange Sherbet (GF)

This sherbet is refreshing and light.

2 cups non-fat milk
1 6-ounce can concentrated frozen orange juice
2 tablespoons honey (optional)

Blend milk, juice and honey or stir until well mixed. Pour into a 9-inch glass oven-proof pie plate and freeze. Place chunks of the frozen orange mixture into a food processor and whip until smooth. Serve immediately. Serves 2 to 3.

POTPOURRI

Appetizers

Your and your guests will be delighted by the exciting and healthy, hot and cold appetizers and snacks in this section. You will find recipes for delicious stuffed mushrooms, vegetarian pate, even baked vegi-tempura, eggplant appetizers, marinated vegetables, Mexican hot snacks and hors d'oeuvres. Since all of these recipes contain either no or low fat, cholesterol or salt, and no sugar, you and your guests can really enjoy them without feeling overly stuffed, or guilty.

Mushrooms Stuffed With Spinach and Herbs

These stuffed mushrooms, flavored with tarragon, make an appealing and delicious low-calorie appetizer, and a fine complement to any meal.

16 large mushrooms (or 30 medium-sized), cleaned and stems removed. Place on a cookie sheet

1 10-ounce package frozen spinach, chopped or leaves, well-thawed, drained and squeezed out gently
1 cup low-fat cottage cheese
¼ medium onion
2 cloves fresh garlic, minced (or ½ teaspoon garlic powder)
¼ cup parsley leaves
1 teaspoon onion powder
¼ teaspoon black pepper
½ teaspoon thyme
½ teaspoon dried dill weed
⅛ teaspoon nutmeg
1/16 teaspoon (or a dash), of cinnamon
¼ teaspoon tarragon
1 tablespoon whole wheat pastry flour

lemon wedges for garnish and added flavor

Rinse mushrooms well, remove stems, and set aside. (Reserve stems for another use.) Puree next 13 ingredients in a blender or food processor. Stuff mushrooms generously and arrange them in a non-stick 10x15-inch jelly roll pan 1 inch apart. Can be held at this point in refrigerator.

Fifteen minutes before serving bake stuffed mushrooms in a 425° oven for 12 to 15 minutes, and serve immediately with a squeeze of lemon on top. Yields 16 hors d'oeuvres.

Mushroom Onion Cheese Hors d'Oeuvres (GF)

1 pound mushrooms, chopped
1 large onion, chopped
2 cloves garlic, minced
¼ teaspoon ground pepper
1 teaspoon thyme

2 tablespoons white wine (optional)

½ cup low-fat cottage cheese

6 slices of whole wheat or Gluten free bread, toasted on one side in oven

sprinkle of paprika for top

Saute first 5 ingredients in a non-stick frying pan slowly until all the moisture is absorbed. Stir occasionally to avoid sticking and burning. Add wine and continue cooking until wine is absorbed. Remove from heat and stir in cottage cheese. Spread mixture on the untoasted side of bread slices. Cut into fours diagonally. Preheat broiler. Arrange hors d'oeuvres in a non-stick 10x15-inch jelly roll pan and sprinkle with paprika. Broil until golden brown, for approximately 5 minutes and serve immediately. Yields 24 hors d'oeuvres.

Garbanzo Bean-Sesame Spread (GF)

This healthy, tasty spread is full of protein and is very easy to prepare.

2 ½ cups cooked garbanzo beans, drained
2 to 4 tablespoons garbanzo bean broth, from above
2 tablespoons lemon juice
½ medium onion, chopped
2 cloves garlic, minced
2 tablespoons chopped parsley
½ small red or green bell pepper

Continues on the next page

2 green onions
½ cup hulled sesame seeds
2 tablespoons sunflower seeds
3 drops Tabasco
1 teaspoon cumin
2 tablespoons apple cider vinegar or red wine vinegar

Grind all ingredients in a food processor or blender until it forms paste. Serve on pieces of pita or crackers, or use as a sandwich spread. Yields 3 ½ cups.

Easy Mexican Hot Snacks with Uncooked Chile Salsa

You can make these tasty snacks in a few minutes.

1 ½ cups low-fat cottage cheese
2 teaspoons onion powder
1 tablespoon whole wheat flour

12 corn tortillas

Uncooked Chile Salsa (see below)

Mix together cottage cheese, flour and onion powder. Spread cottage cheese in the center of each tortilla, top cottage cheese with Uncooked Chile Salsa, and fold tortillas in half. Bake in a 450° oven in a non-stick 10x15-inch jelly roll pan until hot and bubbly. Allow to cool for a few minutes before serving. These appetizers may be cut in half after baking. Serves 6 to 8.

Uncooked Chile Salsa (GF)

1 cup chopped seeded tomatoes
½ cup chopped green onions
¼ cup chopped fresh green chiles (or 1 4-ounce can of diced green chiles)

Mix salsa ingredients together. Store in refrigerator, and use sparingly on Mexican dishes. Yields 2 cups of salsa.

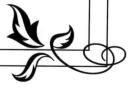

Pimiento Cream Dip (or Spread) (GF)

This makes a delicious spread that is very easy to prepare, and a beautiful salmon color.

2 cups low-fat cottage cheese
1 small, fresh pimiento, chopped; or 2-ounces canned, sliced pimiento
¼ small onion (or 1 teaspoon onion powder)

Blend all ingredients in food processor or blender. Use mixture to stuff celery stalks, as a spread on whole wheat crackers, or as a sandwich spread. Yields 2 cups.

Marinated Vegetables with Herb Dressing (GF)

Enjoy these marinated vegetables as light snacks, or as a salad or appetizer.

2 cups sliced carrots
2 cups cauliflower florets
2 cups broccoli florets
2 cups boiling water

2 cups zucchini slices
8 to 12 mushrooms, cut in half or quarters
1 small onion, sliced thin

1 cup apple cider vinegar
2 tablespoons concentrated apple juice
¼ teaspoon black pepper
2 tablespoons lemon juice
4 cloves garlic
½ teaspoon thyme
½ teaspoon basil
½ teaspoon dill

Continues on the next page

In a medium-sized pot combine the first 4 ingredients. Cook for 3 minutes, rinse in cold water and drain. Place these vegetables in a large mixing bowl. Add raw zucchini, mushrooms and onion. In a smaller bowl mix all remaining ingredients, and pour this dressing over vegetables. Toss well.

Marinate vegetables in refrigerator for a least 4 hours, or longer if possible. Serves 6 to 8.

Oven-Baked Vegi-Tempura Appetizers

These appetizers are very low in calories. You can munch on them to your hearts delight. They taste especially great dipped into Homemade Chili Sauce, or Mickey's Tangy Relish. Leftovers may be eaten cold.

Batter:
2 cups low-fat cottage cheese
2 tablespoons non-fat yogurt

⅔ cup whole wheat flour
1 teaspoon baking soda
1 teaspoon baking powder
6 egg whites
1 tablespoon onion powder
½ teaspoon black pepper
1 teaspoon curry powder
1 teaspoon garlic powder

Whip cottage cheese and yogurt in blender or food processor. Stir in remaining ingredients and blend a moment longer. Pour into a large mixing bowl.

Vegetables:
12 to 18 medium-sized mushrooms, whole
½ medium cauliflower, broken or cut into 12 to 15 florets
2 to 3 large broccoli stalks, cut into 12 to 15 florets

Continues on the next page

Rinse and drain raw vegetables well on a clean dry towel. Using a fork to spear each piece, dip pieces into batter. Shake off excess and arrange pieces in non-stick jelly roll pans. Group mushrooms together on the same cookie sheet since they require less baking time. Do not overcrowd. Bake mushrooms in a 425° oven for 18 to 20 minutes, and bake cauliflower and broccoli for 25 minutes. Appetizers are ready when they are lightly browned. Remove with spatula and serve at once. Yields 36 to 48 hors d'oeuvres.

Eggplant Appetizer for Onion Lovers (GF)

This appetizer has a strong taste of onion. For those fond of onions, this is a marvelous appetizer.

1 medium eggplant, unpeeled, cut in half lengthwise
½ cup water

1 large onion, chopped
3 cloves garlic, minced

3 tablespoons tomato puree
3 tablespoons concentrated apple juice
2 tablespoons red wine vinegar
2 teaspoons cumin
dash of cinnamon

1 teaspoon ground coriander

Place halves of eggplant center-side down in 9x13-inch non-stick baking pan. Pour ½ cup of water around the eggplant, and bake in a 450° oven for 30 minutes or until soft when pressed on. Remove eggplant from oven, peel skin off, and cut into large chunks.

   While the eggplant is baking saute the onion and garlic in a non-stick frying pan until lightly brown. Remove pan from heat. After eggplant is soft, puree it, then add it to the onion mixture in the frying pan. Stir in next 5 ingredients. Simmer for 5 to 8 minutes. Add coriander and refrigerate. Serve cold on Gluten Free crackers or Gluten Free bread or whole grain bread. Serves 6 to 8.

Puffed Potato Appetizers (GF)

These are fun, and good for you too.

Potato Filling:
4 medium boiling potatoes, peeled, cut into quarters
1 ½ cups water

1 large onion, chopped
3 cloves garlic
¼ cup water

½ teaspoon dried parsley flakes
1 teaspoon dill weed
½ teaspoon celery seed
1 teaspoon cider vinegar
¼ teaspoon black pepper
½ cup low-fat cottage cheese

Bring potatoes to a boil, and simmer until potatoes are tender when pierced with a fork. Meanwhile saute onions and garlic in water until onions are soft and lightly browned. Drain potatoes, and puree them with cottage cheese, herbs, vinegar and pepper. Stir in sauteed onions and set aside.

Batter:
2 cups low-fat cottage cheese
2 tablespoons non-fat yogurt

⅔ cup whole wheat flour or Gluten Free flour
1 teaspoon baking soda
1 teaspoon baking powder
6 egg whites
1 tablespoon onion powder
½ teaspoon black pepper
1 teaspoon garlic powder

Continues on the next page

Whip cottage cheese and yogurt in blender or food processor. Add remaining ingredients and blend a moment longer.

To assemble: Fill non-stick muffin tins ½ full with batter, then place 1 heaping tablespoon of potato mixture in center of each muffin tin, and bake in a 350° oven for 25 to 30 minutes. Let Potato Puffs stand for 10 minutes. Remove gently from tins and serve warm.

Note: — It is natural for the puffs to shrink as they cool. Yields 16 to 18 appetizers.

Mushrooms Stuffed with Duxelle and Herbs (GF)

These hors d'oeuvres are winners, and so lean. Your guests will want more than one.

16 large mushrooms (or 30 medium-sized)

1 medium onion, cut in eighths
3 cloves garlic

2 slices whole grain or Gluten free bread, toasted, cut into eighths
½ cup walnut chunks

1 cup low-fat cottage cheese
¼ cup parsley leaves
1 teaspoon onion powder
¼ teaspoon black pepper
½ teaspoon thyme
½ teaspoon dried dill weed
⅛ teaspoon nutmeg
¹⁄₁₆ teaspoon (or a dash) of cinnamon
¼ teaspoon tarragon

sprinkle of paprika for top

Rinse mushrooms well, remove stems, pat caps dry and set aside. Chop stems, onion and garlic in a blender or food processor. Saute this mixture in a non-stick frying pan over low heat until moisture is absorbed.

Continues on the next page

Meanwhile finely chop bread and walnuts in blender or food processor, and place this mixture into a mixing bowl. Blend next 9 ingredients in a blender or food processor. Add this to the bread-nut mixture in the mixing bowl. Mound filling into mushrooms. Arrange them in a non-stick 10x15-inch jelly roll pan 1 inch apart. Sprinkle with paprika and bake in a 425° oven for 12 to 15 minutes. Serve immediately. Makes 16 hors d'oeuvres.

Creamy Cottage Cheese Dip with Green Onions (GF)

This is a tasty, low cholesterol dip for raw vegetables or baked potatoes.

2 cups low-fat cottage cheese
2 to 3 green onions, tops and bottoms cut into pieces for blender

Blend cheese and onions together well. Chill. Yields 2 cups.

Quick Curry Cheese Hors d'Oeuvres (GF)

These hors d'oeuvres are easy to make, delicious and nutritious.

2 cups low-fat cottage cheese
4 teaspoons curry powder
2 teaspoons onion powder
¼ teaspoon black pepper

6 slices whole wheat or Gluten free bread, toasted on 1 side in oven

Heat first 4 ingredients in a non-stick frying pan just until cheese begins to melt.
Spread curry sauce on the untoasted side of bread slices. Cut into fours diagonally. Preheat broiler. Arrange hors d'oeuvres in a 10x15-inch non-stick jelly roll pan, and broil until golden brown, for approximately 5 minutes. Serve immediately. Yields 24 hors d'oeuvres.

Vegetarian Pate (Mock Chopped Liver) (GF)

This tasty spread is cholesterol-free. It tastes a little like chopped liver.

1 large onion, chopped

1 cup ground walnuts
1 10-ounce package frozen string beans, cooked and drained
2 hardboiled egg whites
⅛ teaspoon black pepper
⅛ teaspoon celery seed
¼ teaspoon garlic powder
5 drops Tabasco

Saute onion in a non-stick frying pan until brown, adding a little water as needed to prevent sticking. Puree onion with remaining ingredients in food processor until the consistency of a pate, or chopped liver. Place on serving plate and serve with whole grain or Gluten Free crackers. Serves 6.

BEVERAGES

⊰⊱

In this section you will find exciting and delicious, hot and cold drinks, made without caffeine, fat, cholesterol, salt or sugar. We feel calmer and much more energetic since we "kicked" the caffeine habit of tea and coffee. It took us about one week to withdraw from the habit, and we haven't missed it since. It is far healthier for us to enjoy these amazingly good, wholesome drinks instead. We hope you will enjoy them too.

⊰⊱

Holiday Fat-Free Egg Nog (GF)

This egg nog tastes rich and flavorful, without the egg yolk, cream and sugar that egg nog usually contains. Holiday cheer everyone!

1 cup non-fat milk
1 cup evaporated skimmed milk
2 tablespoons honey
⅛ teaspoon nutmeg
⅛ teaspoon coriander
1 egg white, beaten until very frothy

2 tablespoons brandy or cognac (optional), or 1 teaspoon rum extract

sprinkle of nutmeg and coriander for top

Whip first 6 ingredients in blender. Heat slowly in a non-stick saucepan, stirring occasionally until hot. If liquor is being used, place 1 tablespoon of liquor in each mug, pour hot egg nog into mugs, sprinkle with nutmeg and coriander, and serve at once.

In case the egg nog appears lumpy, blend it for a few seconds in a blender or food processor. Serves 2.

Apple Thirstquencher (GF)

Here is a delicious thirstquencher that's sweetened only with apple juice.

⅓ cup concentrated frozen apple juice, unsweetened

⅔ cup salt-free soda water

ice cubes

Place apple juice in tall glass. Stir in soda until well mixed. Add ice cubes. Serves 1.

Note: — *Salt-free soda is available in most large supermarkets. If it is not available, substitute water or regular soda as desired.*

Grapefruit Thirst-quencher (GF)

This healthy refreshing drink will really quench your thirst.

⅓ cup concentrated frozen grapefruit juice, unsweetened
1 teaspoon honey, optional

⅔ cup salt-free soda water

ice cubes

Mix grapefruit juice with honey in tall glass. Stir in soda until well mixed. Add ice cubes. Serves 1.

Note: – *Salt-free soda is now available in most large supermarkets. If it is not available, substitute water or regular soda as desired.*

Foamy Pineapple-Apple Party Punch (GF)

Whenever we serve this punch, it never fails that guests ask for the recipe. We feel good about serving this healthy punch.

1 48-ounce can of unsweetened pineapple juice
2 12-ounce cans frozen concentrated apple juice
2 large bottles salt-free soda (42 ounces or 1 liter each)
25 to 30 ice cubes

Mix together ingredients in a large punch bowl and serve. Serves 18 to 20.

Hot Carob-Postum Drink (GF)

This satisfying drink contains no caffeine. You can enjoy it morning and night.

1 tablespoon carob powder
½ tablespoon Postum

6 ounces boiling water

6 ounces hot non-fat milk
½ teaspoon dark molasses

Stir boiling water into carob powder and Postum in a large mug. Then add hot milk and molasses. Stir well. Serves 1.

Cold Carob-Postum Drink

In warm weather this drink is great!

1 tablespoon carob powder
1 ½ teaspoons Postum (plain-flavored)
2 tablespoons boiling water

½ teaspoon or 1 teaspoon dark molasses

4 ounces cold non-fat milk

ice cubes to fill a tall glass

ice water, as needed, to fill glass

Place carob powder and Postum in a tall glass. Stir in boiling water and molasses, then add milk, ice cubes and ice water. Stir well. Serves 1.

Caffeine-Free Carob Capuccino (GF)

You'll feel pampered with this rich-tasting delicious drink, and you'll be able to sleep like a baby.

1 tablespoon of carob powder

8 ounces boiling water

¼ cup evaporated skimmed milk
½ to 1 teaspoon dark molasses
dash of cinnamon

Place carob powder in a large cup or mug. Add boiling water, and stir in milk, molasses and cinnamon. Serves 1.

Hot Almond Drink (GF)

For a taste treat try this.

1 cup evaporated skimmed milk
1 cup water
1 tablespoon honey

½ teaspoon pure almond extract
1 teaspoon vanilla

sprinkle of nutmeg on top

Heat milk, water and honey in a small non-stick pan until hot. Add almond and vanilla extracts and pour into cups. Sprinkle nutmeg on top. Serves 2.

Hot Lemonade (GF)

Excellent for colds, sore throats and chills.

1 tablespoon lemon juice (approximately ½ lemon)
1 teaspoon honey
8 ounces boiling water

Place lemon juice and honey in a large mug. Stir in boiling water. Inhale between sips. Serves 1.

Healthful Ginger Root Tea (GF)

This tea is warming and is a good aid for digestion.

4 slices of fresh ginger root, each the size and thickness of a quarter
2 cups water

1 teaspoon honey per cup (optional)

Cook ginger root and water for approximately 5 minutes. Pour into cups. Stir in honey if desired. Serves 2.

CONDIMENTS & RELISHES

Homemade Apple Butter (GF)

Spread this delicious, low-calorie spread on bread, muffins and pancakes.

1 12-ounce jar unsweetened applesauce
½ cup concentrated apple juice
3 teaspoons cornstarch
4 teaspoons cinnamon
¼ teaspoon ginger
pinch of cloves
¼ teaspoon of nutmeg

2 teaspoons vanilla extract

Cook first 7 ingredients in a non-stick saucepan until mixture thickens. Continue to simmer for 5 minutes. Remove from heat, stir in vanilla and store in refrigerator. Yields 2 ½ cups.

Flo's Homemade Orange Marmalade (GF)

This treat is easy to make, and tastes great on breads, muffins and pancakes.

1 cup Cooked Orange Peel, (see chapter on Basics)
½ cup honey
¼ teaspoon coriander
2 tablespoons water

Simmer ingredients very slowly in a small non-stick saucepan for 25 to 30 minutes, stirring occasionally. Store in refrigerator. Yields 1 ½ cups.

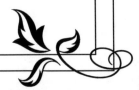

Salt-Free Kosher Dill Pickles (GF)

These pickles taste great, and they take only 10 minutes to prepare. You won't miss the salt.

5 or 6 pickling cucumbers, each cut in 3 or 4 diagonal slices, or into quarters
1 teaspoon dried dill (or 1 tablespoon fresh dill)
2 teaspoons onion powder
½ cup white vinegar
1 cup water
6 cloves of garlic, cut in half

Mix together all the ingredients in a wide-mouthed quart jar with a lid. Cover, and place in refrigerator for 1 or 2 days as desired. Yields 1 quart.

Cranberry Orange Relish (GF)

This relish is great for holiday buffets.

1 pound fresh cranberries, rinsed and drained
½ cup honey
½ cup concentrated orange juice
1 teaspoon ground ginger
grated orange peel of 2 medium oranges, or ¼ cup Cooked Orange Peel (see chapter on Basics)

Cook all ingredients over medium-high heat until cranberries pop, for about 10 minutes. Remove from heat and skim off foam. Serve chilled. Yields 3 cups.

Homemade Catsup (GF)

Use this on Fat-Free Oven-Baked French Fries and enjoy.

2 cups tomato puree
¼ cup white vinegar
2 tablespoons concentrated apple juice

Cook ingredients in saucepan over low heat, stirring occasionally until quantity is reduced down to 1 ½ cups. Store in refrigerator in a glass jar. Yields 1 ½ cups.

Homemade Chili Sauce (GF)

2 cups tomato puree
½ cup onion, finely chopped
2 cloves garlic, minced
1 teaspoon chili powder, or more to taste
¼ cup white vinegar
2 tablespoons concentrated apple juice

Simmer ingredients in a small saucepan over low heat for 1 hour, stirring occasionally until quantity is reduced down to 1 ¾ cups. Store in refrigerator in a glass jar. Yields 1 ¼ cups.

Mickey's Tangy Relish (GF)

Use this relish on lentil-cheese burgers. It's the greatest!

8 tablespoons Homemade Chili Sauce (see above)
2 tablespoons mustard (salt free)
6 drops Tabasco
½ teaspoon cumin
½ teaspoon curry powder

Mix together all the ingredients, and store in the refrigerator. Yields ⅔ cup.

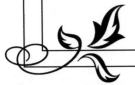

BASIC RECIPES

For your convenience in this section we have grouped together recipes which are called for repeatedly in making other recipes. The Mock Soy Sauce, for example, brings magic to many tofu recipes. The Cooked Orange Peel tastes marvelous in many cakes, breads and muffins. At last you can prepare many Mexican dishes with this great tasting salt and fat free Enchilada Sauce.

You may wish to use the recipes from this section to create a variety of your own favorite entrees, appetizers, salads, desserts and baked goodies. With a little imagination there is no end to the delightful surprises you can come up with.

Mock Soy Sauce (GF)

It took a small stroke of genius for us to create this healthy, salt-free substitute for soy sauce. It tastes great with tofu dishes.

3 tablespoons white vinegar
2 teaspoons dark molasses
¾ teaspoon onion powder
½ teaspoon garlic powder

Mix all ingredients together and serve with brown rice and tofu dishes. Store in refrigerator. Yields ¼ cup.

Cooked Orange Peel (GF)

Use this cooked peel for baking and for making Flo's Homemade Orange Marmalade. It gives cakes, breads, muffins and cookies such a delicious flavor.

peel of 4 to 6 oranges (including white part), cut into pieces
water to top of pot

Cook peel in a 3-quart pot full of water for ½ hour. Drain off water, and rinse peel. Then add fresh water and repeat process. Drain again, add fresh water and soak peel for several hours or overnight. Drain, then chop peel in food processor or blender. Refrigerate, or freeze for use in baking. Yields 1 ½ to 2 cups.

Home-Made Enchilada Sauce (GF)

This easy-to-prepare sauce can be used generously over Mexican casseroles and other Mexican favorites.

1 cup tomato puree
3 cups water
2 teaspoons chili powder
1 tablespoon onion powder
⅛ teaspoon pepper
1/16 teaspoon cayenne
½ teaspoon garlic powder

1 tablespoon potato or cornstarch
2 tablespoons cold water

Cook first 7 ingredients in a 2-quart saucepan over medium heat until sauce comes to a boil. Reduce heat and simmer for 10 minutes. In a cup dissolve starch in water and gradually add in starch, stirring constantly until sauce thickens a little. Yields 1-quart.

Basic Cooked Brown Rice (GF)

This healthy brown rice recipe is easy and foolproof, as long as your are there to turn it off on time.

2 cups raw brown rice, rinsed
5 cups water, Garbanzo Bean Broth or Cauliflower Broth (see chapter on Basics)

Bring rice and water or broth to a boil in a non-stick saucepan. Cook over medium heat covered until water or broth is absorbed, for approximately 35 to 45 minutes. Gently fluff rice with a fork. Yields 5 cups of rice.

Note: — *Use rice in various recipes. Two teaspoons of onion powder may be added if water is used, unless rice is to be used for a sweet or dessert recipe. Yields 5 cups.*

Tender Whole Wheat Crepes

These crepes are great. We use these crepes to make Cheese Blintzes, Blintze Souffle and Apple Crepes.

6 egg whites
½ cup evaporated skimmed milk
1 ¾ cups water

1 ½ cups whole wheat flour

Whisk first 3 ingredients in a large mixing bowl. Add flour, all at once, whisking just until blended. Chill batter for a few hours for more tender crepes. To fry crepes heat a small non-stick frying pan or omelette pan. Lightly grease pan in-between each crepe. Pour a large serving spoon full of crepe batter into the pan. Tilt pan quickly to spread batter. If batter is too thick, add a little more water. Fry crepes over medium heat until top of crepe is dry. Turn for a few seconds, remove from pan, and cool on a clean towel or cloth. Crepes can then be stacked until ready to use. Yields 12 to 14 crepes.

Black Raisin Syrup with Orange Peel and Spices (GF)

Use this syrup over pancakes and in baking cakes and breads in place of honey.

1 cup black raisins
2 cups water
2 tablespoons concentrated apple juice
1 teaspoon coriander
1 teaspoon cinnamon
2 tablespoons Cooked Orange Peel (see chapter on Basics), or 1 tablespoon grated orange
    peel

Bring all of the ingredients to a boil in a medium-sized, non-stick saucepan. Cover, reduce heat to low and simmer for 35 minutes. Cool and then puree mixture in a blender or food processor. Store in refrigerator. Yields 1 cup thick syrup.

Creamy Whipped Cottage Cheese Yogurt Topping (GF)

This is an excellent topping for baked potatoes or a base for dips and salad dressings. Chives, green onions or pimiento can be added.

2 cups low-fat cottage cheese
2 tablespoons non-fat yogurt
1 teaspoon onion powder

Blend all ingredients in blender or food processor until smooth and creamy. Yields 2 ¼ cups.

Non-Dairy Whole Wheat Crepes

These non-dairy crepes can be used for apple or fruit crepes, or for cheese blintzes.

1 cup whole wheat flour or pastry flour
1 ¼ cups cold water
4 egg whites

Whisk ingredients in a mixing bowl until blended. Fry crepes in non-stick omelette pan or small frying pan, lightly greased with a little oil in-between each crepe, until crepe is set on one side. (Crepe will begin to pull away from the edge of pan.) Lift crepe, turn it over, and fry for a few seconds. Remove from pan and cool on a clean towel or cloth. Crepes can then be stacked until ready to use. Yields 12 to 14 crepes.

Note: – If batter is too thick, add a little more water.

Mock Sour Cream (GF)

We found this recipe in the 1973 American Heart Association pamphlet. We omitted the salt. It can be used in various ways and in many recipes.

2 tablespoons non-fat milk
1 tablespoon lemon juice
1 cup low-fat cottage cheese

Blend all ingredients until smooth and creamy. Yields 1 ¼ cups.

Spicy Refried Beans (GF)

You won't miss the salt in these tasty beans. Once the beans are made they can be used in a variety of Mexican dishes, or eaten as a side dish.

1 pound pink or pinto beans (2 ¼ cups)
water to cover

6 cups water

1 medium onion, chopped
3 cloves garlic, minced

2 teaspoons chili powder
1 teaspoon cumin
1 teaspoon oregano
1 cup tomato puree
2 teaspoons red wine vinegar

Bring beans and water to a boil in a large pot and cook beans for 10 minutes. Allow beans to remain in hot water until water cools or overnight. Drain, rinse beans, and return them to pot. Add 6 cups of water. Bring beans to a boil, cover, then reduce heat and simmer beans slowly until tender, for approximately 2 ½ hours.

Meanwhile saute onion and garlic in a large non-stick frying pan. When pan becomes dry, add last 5 ingredients. Stir in cooked beans and simmer beans for a few minutes. Yields 2-quarts of beans.

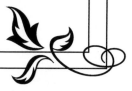

Easy Homemade Non-Fat Yogurt (GF)

This easy-to-prepare, soft-set yogurt is excellent for cooking, baking, and frozen desserts. When we have less than 1 cup left we make a new batch.

½ cup plain low-fat or non-fat yogurt (as a starter)
2 cups non-fat milk, or 1 cup evaporated skimmed milk plus 1 cup water

Mix yogurt and milk together in a small bowl. Cover and let mixture stand in a warm part of kitchen until soft set. This usually takes between 24 and 36 hours, depending on how warm it is in the kitchen. Refrigerate or freeze depending on its use. Yields 2 ½ cups.

Garbanzo Bean Broth (GF)

We use this broth as a stock to enhance soups and rice dishes. Beans can be used in Marinated Bean Salad or Garbanzo Sandwich Filling.

2 cups garbanzo beans, raw
9 cups water

10 cups water
1 large onion, whole (or 1 tablespoon onion powder)
4 cloves garlic, whole (or 1 teaspoon garlic powder)
1 tablespoon dried dill weed
1 teaspoon celery seed
1 tablespoon dried parsley flakes

Bring beans and 9 cups of water to a boil in a large soup pot, and continue to boil for 15 minutes. Remove from heat, and allow beans to remain in hot water until cool or overnight.

Drain, rinse and return beans to pot. Add all remaining ingredients and cook covered on stove until tender for approximately 2 ½ hours, or in a crockpot for 10 hours. Yields 1 ½ to 2-quarts of broth.

Note: — *Store broth in quart jars in refrigerator or freezer until ready to use as base for soups or rice dishes. This broth can also be combined with Cauliflower Broth below to be used as stock for soups and rice dishes.*

Cauliflower Broth (GF)

This broth makes an excellent tasty stock for soups.

1 medium-sized cauliflower, whole
8 cups water
1 medium onion (1 tablespoon onion powder)
2 cloves garlic (or ½ teaspoon garlic powder)
1 teaspoon celery seed
¼ teaspoon ground black pepper
1 teaspoon dill weed
1 tablespoon dried parsley leaves

In a covered soup pot cook the cauliflower with remaining ingredients until tender. Use the broth as a base for soups. It can be stored in quart jars in the refrigerator or freezer until ready for use. Yields 1 ½-quarts of broth.

How to Combine Foods to Boost Nutrition

Grains have certain essential amino-acids, but grains are not complete proteins in themselves. This is also true of beans (or lentils) and of dairy products. However, when grains and beans, or grains and dairy products are eaten together in the same meal, the amino-acids in each group link together to provide a more complete protein. Egg whites, seeds and nuts provide additional protein.

Many of the recipes in this book contain combinations of foods which provide complete protein, such as the two combinations below:

> — grains, cereal, flour, bread, tortillas, potatoes, pasta
> combined with
> cottage cheese, milk, yogurt

> — grains, cereal, flour, bread, tortillas, potatoes, pasta
> combined with
> beans, lentils, peas

Equipment, Pots and Utensils We Use For Cooking and Baking

Food processor and blender. (It is not necessary to buy an expensive model. For many years we used a model which sold for under $50.00)

Pots and Pans:

For frying: non-stick omelette pans, non-stick frying pan

For cooking: non-stick pots of various sizes, enamel pots, stainless steel pots, double boiler, large crockpot

For baking: non-stick cookie sheets and jelly roll pans; non-stick and glass oven-proof baking pans, sizes 9x9-inch and 9x13-inch; 9-inch glass oven-proof pie plates, (with extended fluted-edge if possible)

Electric mixer

Wire whisk

Wooden spoons

Plastic spatulas

Mixing bowls, assorted sizes, of glass and ceramic

Cake tester

TIPS FOR SHOPPING AND COOKING HEALTHY

Foods and Products We Use

Dairy Products: low-fat oraganic (if possible) cottage cheese (1 or 2% fat), hoop cheese (dry curd skim milk cottage cheese), non-fat milk, evaporated skimmed milk, non-fat dry curd cottage cheese, yogurt, buttermilk

Soy Products: Tofu

Eggs: Whites only. We throw the yolks away. It's better to throw them away than to have them clog up your arteries.

Legumes: garbanzo beans (or CiCi beans), lima beans, kidney beans, soy beans, lentils, split peas

Grains: brown rice, buckwheat, whole grain cereals, bran flakes, quinoa, millet

Breads: Gluten free or whole grain bread, pita, salt-free rice cakes, corn tortillas

Flours: whole wheat flour, whole wheat pastry flour, cornmeal, buckwheat flour, rice and almond flour

Pastas: whole wheat and soy pastas, gluten free rice or corn or quinoa pastas

Nuts: raw almonds, walnuts, pecans

Seeds: sunflower seeds, sesame seeds, and seed meals

Bottled Products: salt-free mustard, salt-free catsup, salt-free chili sauce, wine vinegar, cider vinegar, white vinegar, and salt-free soda

Canned Goods: tomato puree, pumpkin, evaporated skimmed milk, crushed pineapple in its own juice

Frozen Products: unsweetened concentrated apple juice and other unsweetened fruit juices, unsweetened fruits, vegetables including chopped spinach, green beans, broccoli, okra, corn and other vegetables

Fresh Fruits: all sorts

Fresh Vegetables: all sorts

Sweeteners: honey, dark molasses, maple syrup and unsweetened apple juice, black raisins and dates

Spices: cinnamon, nutmeg, ginger, cloves, cumin, chili, curry, dill, Italian seasonings, thyme, coriander, cardamom, allspices, tarragon, turmeric, basil, oregano, pepper, cayenne

TIPS FOR FAT-FREE FRYING

Sauteing Onions or Other Vegetables:

Heat non-stick frying pan over medium heat. Add onions or other vegetables and 1 or 2 tablespoons of water. Stir occasionally with a wooden spoon. If onions or vegetables begin to stick, add a little more water, stirring to release all onions from sides and bottom of pan. Repeat this process until onions or vegetables are softened.

Browning Onions or Other Vegetables:

Use the same process as for sauteing onions or other vegetables listed above, except do not add water in the beginning. Stir onions or vegetables occasionally with a wooden spoon. After they brown a little and begin to stick, add a little water and continue to saute until softened.

Frying Pancakes:

Heat a non-stick griddle or large non-stick frying pan. Fry pancakes until brown on both sides.

Reheating Leftovers:

Heat a non-stick frying pan. Add food to be heated. Cover the pan. Turn when hot and brown on one side. Cover and heat on other side for a few minutes until brown. Portions of food can also be reheated in oven.

Making Egg White Omelettes:

Heat a non-stick omelette pan and apply Pam or a tiny amount (approximately ¼ teaspoon) of butter, margarine or oil evenly to bottom and sides of pan. Otherwise the egg whites will stick. We keep ¼ pound of butter in the freezer for occasional use. That lasts us for about one year.

Making Crepes:

Heat a non-stick omelette pan and apply a tiny amount of Pam or oil on a piece of paper towel to the heated pan. Repeat for each crepe. The amount of oil needed for 12 crepes is less than 1 teaspoon. Store oil in refrigerator so it won't turn rancid.

How to Improvise on your own Favorite Recipes

Many recipes can be adapted to low-fat, low-cholesterol, low-salt and sugar-free cooking and baking. Cake recipes are very difficult to improvise on because most cake recipes call for a minimum of one-half cup of butter, shortening or oil, whole eggs, plus a lot of sugar. It has taken a lot of experimentation for us to be able to bake cakes, pies, cookies, breads and muffins the way we do. We are thrilled with the results.

If a recipe calls for fat, such as butter, shortening, margarine or oil, we omit it entirely, except for 1 tablespoon of oil in only a few cake recipes. We substitute liquid such as apple juice, milk, or yogurt in place of the missing fat.

In place of sugar we substitute honey, concentrated apple juice, chopped dates or raisins. We eliminate all salt and replace it with onion powder, garlic powder or herbs and spices. We use carob powder in place of chocolate and additional egg whites to replace egg yolks (which we never use). Low-fat cottage cheese is used as a substitute for other cheeses called for in recipes. Brown rice, whole grains and whole grain flours are used in place of white rice or white flour.

In order to show you how to improvise on your own favorite recipes, below we provide examples of recipes which we have taken and modified to eliminate the fat, cholesterol, salt and sugar. The modified versions, (minus the fat), may require more or less baking time than the original recipe, and/or a different baking temperature. This may require some experimentation on your part. It has taken us years to develop these recipes, and to learn how to modify our own favorite recipes, so be patient.

Baked Custard

Original Recipe Ingredients	Modified Recipe Ingredients
2 ⅔ cups milk	1 ⅔ cups evaporated skimmed milk
1 cup water	
3 eggs	6 egg whites
1 tablespoon whole wheat pastry flour	
1 cup sugar	½ cup honey
1 teaspoon vanilla	1 teaspoon vanilla
dash nutmeg	dash nutmeg

Honey Carrot Cake

Original Recipe Ingredients	Modified Recipe Ingredients
2 cups regular flour	2 cups whole wheat pastry flour
4 eggs 2 tablespoons whole wheat flour	8 egg whites
2 cups sugar	¾ cup honey
1 cup oil ½ cup concentrated apple juice ½ cup water	1 tablespoon oil
2 teaspoons baking soda 1 teaspoon baking powder	1 tablespoon baking soda
1 tablespoon cinnamon	1 tablespoon cinnamon
1 tablespoon nutmeg	1 tablespoon nutmeg
2 teaspoons vanilla	2 teaspoons vanilla
3 cups grated carrots	3 cups grated carrots
1 cup raisins	1 cup raisins
½ cup chopped nuts	½ cup chopped nuts

Creamy Potato Leeks Soup

3 tablespoons butter	(fat omitted)
3 medium leeks	3 medium leeks
6 to 8 stalks celery	8 stalks celery
2 to 3 boiling potatoes	3 boiling potatoes
2 tablespoons chicken bouillon 1 cup water combination of both	1 cup Cauliflower Broth or Garbanzo Bean Broth or

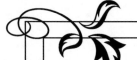

4 cups milk (or half and half)
evaporated skimmed milk and
2 cups water)

3 cups non-fat milk (or 2 cups

salt to taste

(salt omitted)

pinch of cayenne

¼ teaspoon cayenne

black pepper to taste

¼ teaspoon pepper

1 cup grated mozzarella cheese

1 ⅔ cups low-fat cottage cheese

HOW TO STORE FOODS

In order to keep foods as fresh and as pure as possible, we store cooked foods in containers made out of glass (oven-proof when necessary), ceramic, stainless steel or enamel. We avoid plastic, aluminum or other metal containers, since we heard it announced on the news a while back that hard plastic containers can leach chemicals into foods, especially if the foods contain vinegar, lemon, or acid. Particles from aluminum and other metals can also get into the food if foods contain tomato products or other ingredients that react on metal. Before using aluminum foil to cover a large baking dish, we place a layer of wax paper over the food first. Then we apply the aluminum foil over this. The wax paper keeps the food free from being reacted upon by the aluminum foil while it is in the freezer or refrigerator.

A dinner plate, turned upside down makes a good cover over bowls and pie plates, and is safer to use, as well as less expensive, than plastic wrap or aluminum foil. Pies can be stacked easily this way.

We store dry foods such as grains, cereals, flours, raisins, seeds and nuts in the refrigerator to keep them fresh. Wide-mouthed canning jars or empty honey cans with plastic lids make excellent storage containers for dry foods. Wide-mouthed canning jars can be purchased by the dozen in most supermarkets. We do use plastic bags for some smaller items. Dried beans and peas can be stored in jars or cans outside of the refrigerator. Nuts kept for long periods should be frozen.

Products We Avoid

We check all labels and avoid all products containing:

- M.S.G.
- white flour
- white or brown sugar
- salt
- chemical additives or preservatives
- artificial sweeteners – artificial flavorings – artificial coloring
- butter – oil – margarine – mayonnaise
- cream, sour cream, and cream cheese
- whole milk, whole cottage cheese (4% fat), all hard and creamy cheeses
- all foods containing caffeine, such as coffee, decaf, and chocolate

ABOUT THE AUTHORS

Florence and Mickey Bienenfeld have always been at the frontier of health issues, from Mental health and healthy cooking, to yoga, exercise and alternative medicine. Back in the 1970's they were truly considered 'health nuts'. Naturally the culture caught up to them and these trends proved to be, in part, the secrets to long and healthy living. Florence was known to never allow an artificial ingredient into her home, and fed mickey and the three kids with pure and natural ingredients only. As health researched began to show the negative impact of artificial ingredients, processed foods, and some of the dangerous fats, Florence decided to create a series of cookbooks to assist people in living a more healthy and natural life. Mickey and his taste buds, as a spicing specialist , and three kids and many guests who tested the recipes were instrumental in the development of this book. Flo and Mickey's books have sold widely and are now considered as part of the foundation of healthy cooking.

INDEX

A

APPENDIX
- Equipment, Pots and Utensils 191
- How to Combine Foods to Boost Nutrition 191
- How to Improvise on your own Favorite Recipes 196
- How to Store Foods 199
- Products We Avoid 199
- Tips for Fat-Free Frying 195
- Tips for Shopping and Cooking Healthy 193

APPETIZERS
- Creamy Cottage Cheese Dip 169
- Easy Mexican Hot Snacks 163
- Eggplant for Onion Lovers 166
- Garbanzo Bean-Sesame Spread 162
- Marinated Vegetables 164
- Mock Chopped Liver 170
- Mushroom Onion Cheese 162
- Mushrooms Stuffed with Duxelle 168
- Mushrooms Stuffed With Spinach and Herbs 161
- Oven-Baked Vegi-Tempura 165
- Pimiento Cream Dip 164
- Puffed Potato 167
- Quick Curry Cheese 169
- Vegetarian Pate 170

B

BASIC RECIPES
- Basic Cooked Brown Rice 184
- Black Raisin Syrup with Orange Peel and Spices 185
- Cauliflower Broth 189
- Cooked Orange Peel 183
- Creamy Whipped Cottage Cheese Yogurt 186
- Easy Homemade Non-Fat Yogurt 188
- Garbanzo Bean Broth 188
- Home-Made Enchilada Sauce 184
- Mock Soy Sauce 183
- Non-Dairy Whole Wheat Crepes 186
- Spicy Refried Beans 187
- Tender Whole Wheat Crepes 185

BEVERAGES
- Apple Thirstquencher 172
- Caffeine-Free Carob Capuccino 175
- Cold Carob-Postum 174
- Foamy Pineapple-Apple Party Punch 173
- Grapefruit Thirst-quencher 173
- Healthful Ginger Root Tea 176
- Holiday Fat-Free Egg Nog 172
- Hot Almond 175
- Hot Carob-Postum 174
- Hot Lemonade 176

BREADS & MUFFINS
- BREADS
  - Apple Spice 36
  - Cracked Wheat Onion with Oatmeal, Bran, Chile and Cheese 37
  - Fat-Free and Salt-Free Corn 40
  - Homemade Fat-Free Banana 39
  - Pumpkin Raisin 34
  - Raisin Sweetened Whole Wheat Bran 34
- MUFFINS
  - Banana Orange Whole Wheat 32
  - Pumpkin Raisin 34
  - Wholesome Whole Wheat Raisin-Bran 35
  - Whole Wheat Orange Raisin Yeast 38

BREAKFAST & BRUNCH
- Blintze Souffle 7
- Blueberry Pancakes 12
- Buckwheat Hotcakes 10
- Buckwheat Kernel Cereal 5
- Carmelized Apple Pancakes 13
- Custard Noodle Pudding 8
- Divine Apple Crepes 9

- Fat-Free Passover Matza Brei 15
- Fat-Free Passover Pancakes 11
- Flo's Fabulous French Toast 9
- Healthy Seven Grain and Bran Cereal 4
- Hot Cracked Wheat, Oats and Bran Cereal 3
- Individual Cottage Cheese Pancake 12
- Individual Egg White Cheese Omelette 6
- Low-Fat Cheese Blintzes 7
- Non-Dairy Apple Pancakes 10
- Passover Apple-Raisin-Nut Souffle 14
- Pumpkin-Spiced Cereal 4
- Scrambled Egg Whites, Onions & Tomatoes 5
- Stuffed Papaya Halves Indian 3

C

CASSEROLES
- Cheese-Corn-Pimiento-Rice 94
- Cholent 86
- Crockpot Carrot-Sweet Potato Tzimmes 77
- Easy Spinach-Cheese 91
- Eggplant Cheese 82
- Eggplant Parmigiana 60
- Gourmet Mushroom-Cheese 98
- Magnificent Manicotti Marinara 59
- Potato-Cheese 77
- Ratatouille 93
- Spicy Layered Lentil-Rice 80
- Stuffed Cabbage Boats 89
- Succulent Vegetarian Low-Cal Moussaka 94
- Superb Spinach-Cheese Lasagna 57
- Tasty Tamale Pie 74
- Vegetarian Low-Fat Mexican 75
- Vegetarian Low-Fat Mexican Corn and Cheese 72
- Yummy Yam-Meringue 87

CEREALS
- Buckwheat Kernel 5
- Healthy Seven Grain and Bran 4
- Hot Cracked Wheat, Oats and Bran 3
- Pumpkin Spice 139

CONDIMENTS & RELISHES
- Cranberry Orange 179
- Flo's Homemade Orange Marmalade 178
- Homemade Apple Butter 178
- Homemade Catsup 180
- Homemade Chili Sauce 180
- Mickey's Tangy Relish 180
- Salt-Free Kosher Dill Pickles 179

CREPES
- Divine Apple 9
- Low-Fat Cheese Blintzes 7
- Mountain of Florentine 61
- Non-Dairy Whole Wheat 186
- Tender Whole Wheat 185

CUSTARD

D

DESSERTS
- CAKES
  - Almond Roll 126
  - Carob Angel 123
  - Carob Fruit and Spice 120
  - Carob-Honey 117
  - Carob Roll 122
  - Fruit Sweetened Apple 116
  - Giant Apple Party 114
  - Healthy Banana 125
  - Honey-Bunny Carrot 118
  - Honey Holiday Health Fruit 121
  - Old World Plum Custard 119
  - Pumpkin Spice 113
  - Viennese Apple 113
- CHEESECAKES
  - Low-Cal Honey Cheese 128
  - Strawberry 127
  - Tall and Fluffy 129
- COBBLER
  - Party Apple 130
- COOKIES
  - Almond 137
  - Carrot and Raisin Chews 136
  - Carrot Dessert Squares 132
  - Coconut Haystacks 133
  - Cooked Honey Oatmeal 142
  - Crispy Carob 134

- Date-Carob Brownies 138
- Date-Raisin-Oat-Bran 141
- Light Date-Nut 134
- Munchy Mandelbrot 137
- Oatmeal-Raisin Chews 131
- Puffed Wheat Crisps 141
- Pumpkin Cereal Spice Chews 139
- Raisin Sweetened Carob Brownies 132
- Spicy Pumpkin Cereal 140
- CUSTARD
  - Tofu Custard 143
- FROSTINGS
  - Creamy Cheese Walnut 118
  - Fluffy Carob 117
- FRUIT
  - Brandied Poached Pear Halves 143
  - Pears Poached with Coriander 144
  - Spicy Baked Apples 144
- MUFFINS
  - Dark Moist Bran 146
- PIES
  - Baked Vanilla Custard 149
  - Blueberry Cheese 148
  - Crustless Pumpkin 149
  - Custard Bread 150
  - Pineapple Cheese 147
  - Quick Apple 146
  - Tofu-Banana-Pineapple 148
- PUDDINGS
  - Apple-Custard Delight 151
  - Brown Rice-Raisin Pudding 151
- SAUCES & GLAZES
  - Blueberry 128
  - Honey Vanilla 145
  - Strawberry 128, 155
- SOUFFLES
  - Fluffy Carob 153
  - Pineapple-Lemon 152
- YOGURT, FROZEN
  - Easy Fat-Free Soft Orange Sherbet 158
  - Pineapple Creamy Soft 156
  - Soft Blueberry-Banana 156
  - Soft Grape-Banana 157
- Soft Meringue Shell Filled with Strawberry Banana 154
- Spiced Apple Soft 157

E

EGGS
- Baked Mushroom Omelette 66
- Fat-Free Passover Matza Brei 15
- Individual Cheese Omelette 6
- Scrambled with Onions & Tomatoes 5

M

MAIN COURSES
- Baked Mushroom Omelette 66
- Baked Potatoes Stuffed with Cheese 69
- Cheese-Corn-Pimiento-Rice Casserole 94
- Cheese-Onion Souffle 76
- Cheesy Whole Wheat Shells 65
- Chili-Bell Pepper Quiche 78
- Cholent 86
- Colorful Curried Vegetables 107
- Crockpot Carrot-Sweet Potato Tzimmes 76, 77
- Crustless Zucchini Quiche 97
- Easy Potato Pancakes 92, 102
- Easy Spicy Mexican Rice-Cheese Bake 72
- Easy Spinach-Cheese Casserole 91
- Eggplant Cheese Casserole 82
- Eggplant Parmigiana 60
- Fabulous Low-Fat Fettucine Alfredo 63
- Fast Taco Salad 71
- Fettucine Primavera 64
- Flo's Farmers Chop Suey 101
- Gourmet Mushroom-Cheese Casserole 98
- Kasha with Mushrooms, Walnuts, and Onions 83
- Leek and Cheese Quiche 79
- Lentil Roast 98
- Luscious Lentil Burgers 100
- Magnificent Manicotti Marinara 59
- Mexican Tostadas 73
- Mountain of Crepes a la Florentine 61
- Nachos Supreme 69

- Oriental Tofu-Vegetable Delight 101
- Oven-Baked Lima Bean-Potato Stew 86
- Pimiento-Chile Quiche 96
- Potato-Cheese Casserole 77
- Potato Pudding 92
- Ratatouille 93
- Rice-Nut Loaf 108
- Scrambled Tofu Jalapeno 103
- Scrumptuous Spinach Soy Burgers 90
- Spicy Layered Lentil-Rice Casserole 80
- Spicy Stuffed Acorn Squash 92
- Steamy Baked Potatoes with Broccoli 88
- Stuffed Bell Peppers with Mushrooms 106
- Stuffed Cabbage Boats 89
- Succulent Vegetarian Low-Cal Moussaka 94
- Superb Spinach-Cheese Lasagna 57
- Tasty Tamale Pie 74
- Thanksgiving Vegi Turkey Loaf 84
- Tofu "Liver" Steak 105
- Tofu "Pepper Steak" 102
- Vegetarian Low-Fat Mexican Casserole 75
- Vegetarian Low-Fat Mexican Corn and Cheese Casserole 72
- Vegi Bean and Cheese Enchiladas 104
- Vegi Chili Beans 67
- Whole Wheat Spinach Noodles 57
- Yummy Yam-Meringue Casserole 87

N

NOODLES & PASTA
- Cheesy Whole Wheat Shells 65
- Fabulous Low-Fat Fettucine Alfredo 63
- Fettucine Primavera 64
- Superb Spinach-Cheese Lasagna 57
- Whole Wheat Spinach 57

P

PANCAKES
- Blueberry Pancakes 12
- Buckwheat 10
- Carmelized Apple 13
- Fat-Free Passover 11

- Individual Cottage Cheese 12
- Non-Dairy Apple 10

POTATOES
- Baked Stuffed with Cheese 69
- Easy Pancakes 92, 102
- Oven-Baked French Fries 105
- Pudding 92

Q

QUICHES
- Chili-Bell Pepper 78
- Crustless Zucchini with Dill 97
- Leek and Cheese with Herbs 79
- Pimiento-Chile 96

R

RICE
- Basic Cooked Brown 184
- Fancy Wild and Brown 108
- Spanish 68

S

SALADS & DRESSINGS
- DRESSINGS
  - Creamy Yogurt 43
  - Easy Vinaigrette 50, 51
  - Flo's French Herb 45
  - Lemon Yogurt 46
  - Non-Fat Green Yogurt 49
  - Orange Yogurt 53
  - Quick Tomato Salad 44
  - Rice Vinegar Mustard 48
  - Tangy Salad 49
  - Yogurt-Sesame Seed 50
- SALADS
  - Carrot-Raisin-Celery 53
  - Crunchy Cauliflower Cucumber 43
  - Cucumber with Pimientos 54
  - Marinated Bean with Pimiento 46
  - Marinated Cucumber 52
  - Marinated Garbanzo Beans 45
  - Marinated Tangy Beet 52
  - Marinated Vegetable 50
  - Middle Eastern Eggplant 43
  - Pineapple Cole Slaw 48

- Red Cabbage Slaw 47
- Tofu Jalapeno 51
- Winter Fresh Fruit 46

SAUCES

- Cooked Chili 70
- Home-Made Enchilada 184
- Hot Salsa 74
- Italian Tomato 57
- Marinara Sauce 59
- Mild Chile 71
- Mushroom Sauce 99
- Quick Curry Cheese 108
- Salsa Fresca 57
- Spicy Cumin-Mustard 81
- Spicy Spanish 66
- Sweet and Sour 90

SOUFFLE

- Blintze Souffle 7
- Cheese-Onion 76
- Passover Apple-Raisin 14

SOUPS

- Beet Borscht with Boiled Potatoes 30
- Cold Cucumber-Dill 23

- Creamy Cauliflower 33
- Creamy French Onion 24
- Creamy Lentil-Potato 19
- Creamy Potato-Leeks 30
- Creamy Tomato 28
- Easy Lentil-Vegetable 26
- Easy Lima Bean 26
- Easy Split Pea 25
- Great Gazpacho 31
- Hearty Lentil-Barley 29
- Mushroom Barley Bean 22
- Quick Spinach-Cheese 32
- Thick Indian Lentil 27
- Thick Minestrone 21
- Thick Spicy Lentil 20

T

TOFU

- "Liver" Steak 105
- Oriental Vegetable Delight 101
- Pepper Steak 102
- Scrambled Tofu Jalapeno 103